The Alzheimer's Spouse

Finding the Grace to Keep the Promise

Mary K. Doyle

in extenso

The Alzheimer's Spouse
Finding the Grace to Keep the Promise
Mary K. Doyle

Edited by Michael Coyne
Cover design and typesetting by Courter & Company

Cover images by
Eshma / Shutterstock.com
d1sk / Shutterstock.com

An In Extenso book published by ACTA Publications, 4848 N. Clark Street, Chicago, IL 60640, (800) 397-2282, www.actapublications.com

Library of Congress Catalog Number: 2019933596
ISBN: 978-0-87946-971-9
Printed in the United States of America by Total Printing Systems
Year 29 28 27 26 25 24 23 22 21 20 19
Printing 12 11 10 9 8 7 6 5 4 3 2

 Text printed on 30% post-consumer recycled paper

THE PROMISE

"I, ___, take you, ___, to be my husband/wife.
I promise to be true to you in good times and in bad,
in sickness and in health.
I will love and honor you
all the days of my life."

Books by Mary K. Doyle

༄

The Alzheimer's Spouse

Fatima at 100, Fatima Today

Grieving with Mary

Hans Christian Andersen, Illuminated by the Message

The Rosary Prayer by Prayer

Mentoring Heroes

Navigating Alzheimer's

Saint Theodora and Her Promise to God

Seven Principles of Sainthood

Young in the Spirit

Contents

A NOTE ON PRONOUNS AND VERBS

In my effort to maintain a conversational tone in this book,
I go back and forth between referring to "our" spouses
(plural), meaning each of our spouses or all of our spouses,
and "your" or "my" spouse (singular), meaning your spouse
or my husband, Marshall. This sometimes causes an awkward
sentence construction. If I have been inconsistent in the use
of pronouns or verbs, please forgive me.
I know you will.

Until Death Do Us Part

For most couples—like you and your spouse and like my husband and me—the wedding was not taken lightly. Preparation for the event consumed all our thoughts (and budgets) for months. We strived to present our best physical self, losing weight or otherwise fussing over our appearance. From designing the invitations to shopping for the perfect dress or tux, we agonized over every detail of the ceremony: the flowers, the photographs, the reception, the menu, and—finally—the perfect honeymoon. We also prepared spiritually, striving to comprehend the magnitude and the holiness of our vow to marry our very life to that of another in a faithful and faith-filled way.

We all knew from the start, of course, that we began our marriage with a covenant, an agreement that would bind us with our spouse through "the good times and the bad times." Few of us, however, reflected much about the implications of the promise to take responsibility to care physically and emotionally for each other, as we confidently and proudly proclaimed, "in sickness and in health, until death do us part." We were young (or at least younger than we are now). We were beginning a joyful new life. We realized there would be unhealthy days somewhere in the future, even expected them. But we could never have anticipated the terrorist known as Alzheimer's disease, which may even have been an uninvited guest at our wedding. It was at Marshall's and mine.

Alzheimer's sneaks into the brains of its victims and can wreak havoc for ten or even twenty years before anyone really begins to notice. By the time we're aware of its presence, the disease has already caused irreversible damage. In addition to sucking the life out of its victims, it torments all those around them—especially, and most poignantly, their spouse or life partner. If you think you have a good chance of being spared from developing Alzheimer's or caring for someone who does, you should think again. More than 5.8 million Americans are living with the disease in 2019, and 50 million are stricken worldwide. A new case is discovered once a minute, about the time you have spent reading these opening pages. Each of these individual sufferers requires three to five caregivers. Alzheimer's is the sixth leading cause of death, claiming more lives than breast and prostate cancer combined. And among the top killers it's the only disease that cannot be prevented, slowed, or cured.

Whether we know anyone with dementia, or have it ourselves, we still must pay heavily for it. Alzheimer's is the most expensive disease in the nation. Few families can afford the exorbitant cost of care for the sometimes decades-long duration of the disease. Caregivers have no choice but to turn to the American taxpayer with what's left of the bill when their own resources are exhausted. The cost to our nation for dementia care in 2019 is estimated at $290 billion, about equal to the annual interest we pay on the nation's crushing 21 trillion national debt. And those numbers are rapidly climbing as baby boomers join the age group most at risk of being diagnosed with Alzheimer's. More than 10,000 Boomers turn 65 every day.

Those of us who already have a loved one with Alzheimer's know the heartache of watching someone so dear to us disappear before our eyes. The disease slowly and methodically claims a little more of them mentally and physically every day, day after day, year after year. Some go more quickly, others live decades, but the average person with Alzheimer's disease lives eight to ten years after diagnosis. It is an agonizing process to witness.

✓ WHAT WE CAN DO...

- Stay informed by reading books and pamphlets on Alzheimer's and other dementias.
- Participate in Alzheimer's research and funding through donations, walks, and distribution of information.
- Be aware of those around you with Alzheimer's disease and support their caregivers.

Alzheimer's in the Marriage

Even the most stable of marriages can be a roller coaster of events, hurdles, and emotions. As a couple vowed to one another for life, we share our celebrations and failures, our shining moments, and the ones we'd rather not see dredged up. Home, family, work, play—we build a life together. It's not perfect. But it's ours.

And then Alzheimer's pops its ugly head into the mix. Confounding symptoms warn us that a dangerous intruder has crept into our spouse's brain and is slowly annihilating it, neuron by neuron. In fact, it has undoubtedly been lurking there for some time. It's likely to have been taking hold for a decade or two.

We strategize, form a defense, and surge ahead. We fight side-by-side, or more correctly, we fight for our loved one as this most formidable opponent marches on, overtaking our spouse's brain until too many cells are left dead or blocked. We fight the hard fight. We never give up. But Alzheimer's always wins.

We provide the best care we can for our loved ones. We help them through the early course of the disease, fully aware that it cannot end well. There is, as of this writing, no cure. We can only assist our spouses in living as fully as possible until they draw their last breath. After all, we promised to care for them in sickness and health, until death does us part.

This book is written for and dedicated specifically to couples struggling with Alzheimer's, because of the insidious way the disease destroys this most important relationship. In my professional life as an author and speaker, I advocate for everyone touched by Alzheimer's, particularly family caregivers. Everyone in this fight is struggling. But caring for a spouse is a unique predicament, unlike caring for a parent, a sibling, or a friend, because we are tied to our spouse on so many levels: financial, psychological, emotional, sexual, the choice of where we make our home, the turns we take in our careers, the hopes we have for the future and the tears we have shed together in the past. All our lives our personal energy is funneled into making a success of our marriage. But once this Alzheimer's intrudes into a marriage, we find ourselves joined to someone who can no longer fully participate in that relationship, often for many years, a person whose declining health means a continuous and predictable stream of losses for both of us.

Suspended in a perpetual state of grief and mourning, we recover from one dramatic change only to encounter the next. We helplessly watch the steady devastation of our spouse. It is an agonizing position to be in.

While I use the terms "married" and "spouse" throughout this book, please know that I'm including all life partners. Whether married five, ten, fifty years, or not at all; or married for the first, second, third or more times, I am referring to two people who live together in a committed relationship, people who have a bond that endures through the good times and the bad.

Alzheimer's is an especially trying disease because of its intensity and duration. It's a disease that affects every function of the body for years. Little by little it breaks its victim down mentally and physically, and may take many years—sometimes decades— to finish its ugly work.

Our loved one may experience periods of little change—plateaus, little downward steps—where they remain stable for a while. During some periods they may present symptoms that are more manageable than are others. But their condition never improves. Only ever downward. Once Alzheimer's claims a victim, it never lets go.

Alzheimer's is a disease that attacks the spousal caregiver as well as its principal victim. Primary caregiving to a loved one with Alzheimer's is an overwhelming responsibility in what feels like an altered universe. The chronic stress of providing care, of enduring the confusion, the repetition, the sorrow, the inevitable loss, can tax our own immune system, putting our own health at great risk.

Our spouses will say and do some very bizarre things. They can be moody and irrational, especially if they experience what is known as sundown syndrome, which often produces a higher level of confusion late in the day. Previously easy-going, they may now burst into anger with little or no provocation. Once strong and independent, they cling to us. As soon as we think we understand them, they abruptly do an about-face.

Alzheimer's, ever the masochist, periodically teases us with a glimpse of our spouse's old self, only to take it away again until some random date we can't predict. A fond memory arises, and we celebrate it together. But the moment is brief, so brief, and suddenly vanishes once again. Every time it happens, we indulge ourselves in the hope that they are getting better. Every time, we are left frustrated and longing for more.

And this fleeting glimpse of our spouse before the disease struck can even happen very near the end. Just prior to death, some people with dementia show signs of what is known as "terminal lucidity," a moment when a brain ravaged with dementia emits one last clear thought before death. The momentary gift is both joyful and heartbreaking.

More painful are the occasions when our spouses become conscious that they are forgetting us and are having difficulty remembering everything they lived for. Panic streaks across their face as they beg us to explain why they can't remember. Those terrifying moments are the hardest for both of us to bear.

We no longer fully understand this person we married or what is really happening to them. Things become so twisted that we may wonder whether *we* aren't the one's losing *our* minds. Our spouse and their needs change so quickly. And we are often so tired, too tired to handle it all. Our new role as caregiver to a spouse with dementia is physically, emotionally, and financially exhausting, and we don't have our go-to person, our rock, our spouse, to lean on.

Unlike children, step-children, other relatives, or friends, spouses can't just get up and leave. We need to think for both ourselves and our spouses every minute of every day and all night long. If they appear to be uncomfortable, we need to figure out what is wrong (they aren't likely to be able to tell us) and how to help. We become so much more than their marital partner at this point. We have become their everything.

✔ WHAT WE CAN DO...

- Rest. Sleep is medicine. Always strive to get a good night's sleep. Hire an overnight caregiver if necessary.
- Appreciate the periods of slow change.
- Vent. Find a counselor with whom to honestly share your feelings.

We're in This Together

Our marriage vows are tested to the max by the assault Alzheimer's makes on our marriage. We promised to love and honor one another until death. Alzheimer's pushes us to the brink in living these vows. The responsibility to maintain a successful marriage in all its aspects shifts in one direction, to our weary shoulders: love, friendship, generosity, respect, patience, loyalty, play time, security, support, trust, open communication, transparency, sharing of a sacred space, humor, compromise. All fall to the Alzheimer's spouse. The imbalance weighs heavily on us.

I know this because my husband, Marshall Brodien, magician, creator of TV Magic Cards and magic products, and portrayer of the beloved character Wizzo from Chicago's Bozo show, is a victim of Alzheimer's disease. I am not a therapist. I'm an author and speaker with a master's degree in Pastoral Theology, writing from personal experience and exhaustive research. I understand all too well what it is to be married to someone with this disease.

I've been privileged to meet many Alzheimer's spouses since I began speaking on the topic of Alzheimer's and writing my book, *Navigating Alzheimer's: 12 Truths About Caring for Your Loved One.* My readers' heartfelt reactions to my book, responses to my blog posts and Facebook page, and their compelling stories have touched me deeply. They are sometimes pained and raw, often awe-inspiring, always insightful. I appreciate every one of them, empathize deeply with what they are going through, and am humbled by their generosity in sharing their experiences with me.

We spouses and primary caregivers to a loved one with Alzheimer's' and other dementias are an isolated, overlooked, perhaps even marginalized group. As the person with Alzheimer's life becomes smaller, so does ours. This is particularly true if there is no one we trust (or can afford to pay) to take on the serious demands of caring for our loved one. Most of us are seniors ourselves at the onset of the disease, and especially by the end of this journey. After caring for someone so intensely for so long, we have little to give to anyone or anything else, including ourselves. Few of us survive the journey intact, unbruised, undiminished.

I am twenty years younger than my husband, Marshall. Although I am now a senior myself and have endured several care-related illnesses since our ordeal began, our age difference makes me younger and somewhat healthier than most people experiencing Alzheimer's ravages in their marriage. Because of this, I feel it is my obligation to speak out on behalf of those who cannot.

I want to raise awareness, in these chapters, about the many ways Alzheimer's disease tests our marriage vows and robs us of the peace and happiness we expected to have in our golden years. We are alive, we are together, but this disease intrudes in every facet of our lives.

So much of our marital relationship is sorely tested. So many of those vows we made all those years ago are put on the line. Could a person be made more acutely aware of what it means to love and serve our spouse faithfully, in sickness and in health, through richer and poorer, until death do us part?

My hope in writing this book is to offer insights gained from years of personal reflection about the predicament of the Alzheimer's spouse, and bring to the table practical suggestions about caring not just for our loved one, but for the relationship we both worked so hard to build. If nothing else, may every reader gain comfort from knowing that he or she is not alone. I understand. I know what you are going through, and a lot of others—I have met so many wonderful people in my speaking engagements—are right there with us.

You may find what follows frank and disturbing. The simple reality is that this is an ugly disease. It is deeply disheartening on so many levels. Our loved one is methodically being destroyed right before our eyes. And there is seemingly little we can do to help them.

We still may embrace a few tender moments as we attend to our beloved spouse. We share the fears of what we are experiencing and what so surely lies ahead. We savor every moment of joy, fully appreciating that the end can come at any second, not necessarily death, but rather the end of our spouse's ability to share some small part of themselves with us once again. We experience so many little deaths. Each moment, every smile, touch, and loving word becomes more precious than we ever imagined.

However, there's no denying this is a tough road to tread. Please keep in mind as you march through your day that you are not alone. Look around for friends and family who love you. Know that organizations such as the Alzheimer's Association are desperately trying to help. And remember that I hold you close in prayer.

✔ WHAT WE CAN DO...

- Mourn what is lost and move on.
- Know that the things you are doing are acts of compassion, however little they may seem to be appreciated.
- Refer to the Alzheimer's Association website (www.alz.org) for helpful information, contacts, and resources.

In Sickness and in Health

Perhaps the most basic promise in a marriage is the vow to care for one another in sickness and in health. When two healthy adults join in matrimony, it's difficult to fathom the consequences of a prolonged illness. Long-term illness happens to other people, right? Old people. And we'll never grow old, will we? But old we do get, and the older we get the more we are confronted by the reality of this vow.

When Marshall and I met, I realized our ages at that time (59 and 39), and the 20-year age difference between us, would probably result in me caring for him at some point. But he appeared strong and healthy, so I never guessed how soon he would be dependent on me for his daily care, never imagined that his health problems would consume our marriage, or that it would be because of a failing mind, and not an overtly physical ailment.

We've now had more years together with Alzheimer's than without. Alzheimer's was nowhere on my radar back in 1995 when I was falling in love with the most wonderful man I'd ever met. A strong and funny man. A man I knew would be kind to me. Like most people, I knew very little about the disease back then. Circumstances have since made me an expert.

I'm regularly asked what has been the hardest part of dealing with Alzheimer's. My honest answer has to be: all of it! There are no easy pieces once Alzheimer's enters your life. Every stage presents a wide range of challenges. Every day brings sorrow.

The beginning was overwhelming, in large part because I didn't yet understand what was happening. The behaviors we at first witness can be quite puzzling. As with most victims of the disease, we sought answers for nearly three years before we received a final diagnosis and understood the culprit to be Alzheimer's.

Because Alzheimer's is a progressive disease, there are continual changes and small losses to adapt to all along the way. There's no cure, no turning back. Every day, I lose a little more of my husband. Every day I experience another small loss. And of course, I have to live with little idea of what comes next and the question of how and when it all will end.

I know firsthand what other spousal caregivers are going through. I know about the long days and sleepless nights, the messy cleanups, hurtful remarks, and terrifying moments of wandering, sundowners, and falls. I know about the isolation and loneliness. And I certainly know of the need for unlimited patience and compassion.

I am not exaggerating when I tell you that caring for Marshall alone for nearly a decade brought me close to death. The intense round-the-clock care he required and the stress I found myself under led to grave failures in my own health. I finally was forced to accept our doctor's repeated advice and place Marshall in a memory care community.

The move relieved me of the 24/7 demands, but it did not eliminate my responsibility to oversee Marshall's care. I continue to consider myself a caregiver; but now I am part of a team. My husband is always on my mind. I visit or speak with him every day, talk to the staff at his home, and review his condition with his medical team. I spend hours on the phone with insurance companies and medical care providers. I drive Marshall to appointments outside his residence, monitor his personal needs, and ensure that he is happy and well-groomed. Regardless of where my husband has gone, whatever shell of him endures, he remains the center of my life.

✔ WHAT WE CAN DO...

- Congratulate yourself on every accomplishment. Even the little ones. It will help you to recognize and appreciate all the vital things you do.
- Accept that change is a part of this disease. There is no status quo.
- Arm yourself with knowledge, so that you can be confident that whatever decisions you make, you have made them with the best information available.

The Basics of Dementia

Dementia is a neurocognitive disorder that describes a whole family of symptoms including mental confusion, memory loss, disorientation with time and space, intellectual impairment, inability to learn new things, and repetition.

Psychologists now describe more than 200 forms of dementia. Some symptoms of dementia are common. Some are more specific to a particular disorder. Alzheimer's is the most common. Others include vascular dementia, Lewy body, frontotemporal dementia, Pick's disease, and normal pressure hydrocephalus. Some forms of dementia can be associated with diseases such as Creutzfeldt-Jakob disease (Mad Cow), Wernicke-Korsakoff Syndrome (often caused by alcoholism), Huntington's, and Parkinson's.

It's not unusual for one person to have a combination of dementias. For example, after a stroke, some people develop both vascular dementia and Alzheimer's. Other individual health factors can also modify a victim's behavior and the particular course of their illness.

Alzheimer's sufferers usually present with the symptoms typical of dementia—memory loss, mental confusion, disorientation, intellectual impairment, inability to learn new things, and repetition—in addition to symptoms quite specific to Alzheimer's. These symptoms include depression, irritability, hallucinations, and paranoia.

Alzheimer's is not a part of normal aging, but nearly half of all 80-year-olds have some form of dementia. One in three seniors dies with it.

Alzheimer's comes in two different forms: early-onset and late-onset. While the effects are similar in each, they differ in both the cause and the person's age when the disease reveals itself.

Late-onset, the most common, occurs in people 65 years of age and older. The changes to the brain cause symptoms to arise over an extended period, often decades. Scientists aren't entirely certain of the root cause. It is believed to be due to a combination of environmental, lifestyle, and genetic factors—particularly the apolipoprotein E (APOE) gene. As with much of what we know about Alzheimer's, confusion about the role of APOE remains. Carriers of the gene may never get Alzheimer's, and many develop the disease without it.

Early-onset Alzheimer's claims much younger people. Some of these victims have been diagnosed as early as in their 20s.

While fewer than 10% of all cases of Alzheimer's are of this type, that's still 570,000 Americans. People with early-onset Alzheimer's tend to show more physical change to the brain, and the disease is often linked to genetic components.

Alzheimer's kills. Although some treatments are proving to help alleviate symptoms, as of this writing we have no cure. Many people with the disease find the quality of their life is improved for several years with prescription medications, a healthy diet, exercise, and some simple efforts at behavior modification.

Alzheimer's symptoms are believed to be caused by a progressive accumulation of beta-amyloid plaques, protein fragments that form between neurons in the brain, and tangles, twisted strands of protein in the neurons. These proteins prevent proper communication of impulses through the nerve fibers. They block messages and destroy the brain cells. And as neurons die, the abilities to talk, think, and reason diminish. In the end, even simple acts like swallowing and breathing can be a challenge.

The progression of the disease will differ from one person to another because of individual preexisting conditions, age, lifestyle, and personality. However, we do see many commonalities in the progression of the disease.

In the early stages, symptoms are usually subtle. We notice our spouses misplacing items, repeating their thoughts, struggling to express themselves, and having trouble performing tasks they previously accomplished with ease. Persistent moodiness may also be evident. Our spouses may have changed from a gentle, happy person to one who is depressed and easily irritated.

Symptoms become more noticeable in the middle stages. This is often when the disease is first recognized and diagnosed. Our spouses begin forgetting even details of their own personal history, their address, and the current date. They may be paranoid and delusional. Repetitive behavior, such as picking at themselves or wringing their hands, is common.

Our spouses may confuse day and night—experiencing restlessness and wandering about the house at night while sleeping during the day. Dressing appropriately is often a challenge. Their wardrobe choices can be eccentric, like wearing multiple tops or mixing daytime and bed clothes. Bladder and bowel movements may be harder to control.

In the final stages, more assistance is needed with even the simplest activities of daily living: bathing, dressing, toileting, and eating. Their ability to communicate will also fail. And they likely are unaware of their surroundings or our presence. Continuous care is required. This stage can be quite lengthy, comprising as much as 40% of the duration of Alzheimer's symptoms.

The stress of Alzheimer's on the body makes our spouses more vulnerable to infections. Keeping them clean is vital, which often excites resistance. They aren't likely to care if they lose bladder control and wet their clothes. Undressing, cleaning them, and re-dressing is more fuss than they want to go through, particularly since they are unable to correctly regulate their body temperature and are chilled when naked.

If our spouses do not die from another illness, such as cancer, stroke, or heart failure, they will pass away from infection, aspiration pneumonia, or weight loss. Reaching the final stages of decline may take anywhere from a few years to a few decades, depending on other health conditions and the age at which they developed the disease.

In addition to genetics and family history, some of the risk factors of Alzheimer's include cardiovascular disease, high blood pressure, diabetes, smoking, obesity, depression, limited physical activity, a fatty or sugary diet, traumatic brain injury, and Down syndrome. Other conditions thought to increase risk may include immune system malfunctions, endocrine disorders, slow-acting viruses or bacteria, and vitamin deficiencies, especially Vitamin D. Hearing loss is a common fellow-traveler, although researches are still studying whether it is a mere symptom of Alzheimer's or itself a significant contributor to cognitive decline.

Almost two thirds of American seniors with Alzheimer's are women. This has long been considered to be because women live longer than men, but a recent study has shown that it may be the result of the influence of hormones. A woman over sixty is twice as likely to develop Alzheimer's disease as breast cancer.

Alzheimer's symptoms are often initially undetected because they are so easily attributed to aging, lack of sleep, stress, or medications. Even doctors may not pick up on the clues of decline for quite some time. Years may pass before we realize what is truly wrong, and by then, much destruction has taken place in the brain.

If you suspect your spouse may be showing signs of Alzheimer's, review the following Alzheimer's Association guideline. If symptoms are evident, schedule an appointment with your doctor for a medical evaluation.

Early Signs of Alzheimer's Disease

1. Memory loss that disrupts daily life, such as forgetting recent information and significant dates and events.

2. Challenges in planning or solving problems, such as trouble preparing a meal or balancing a checkbook.

3. Difficulty completing familiar tasks, such as driving to a familiar location, managing a familiar work task, or remembering the rules of a favorite game.

4. Confusion with time and place, such as not knowing the day or season. Forgetting where they are or how they got there is another symptom.

5. Trouble understanding visual images and spatial relationships, such as having difficulty reading, judging distance, and determining color or contrast.

6. New difficulty with words in speaking or writing, such as having trouble following or joining in a conversation and using words correctly.

7. Misplacing items and losing the ability to retrace steps, such as putting things in unusual places or losing things. They also may accuse others of stealing and become paranoid.

8. Diminished judgement, like becoming reckless with money or grooming themselves carelessly.

9. Withdrawal from work or social activities, such as declining to participate in their usual social activities, work projects, or sports.

10. A diminished sense of smell. Any person who cannot identify the aroma of peanut butter waved under their nose when they are blindfolded should be tested.

11. Changes in mood or personality, becoming confused, suspicious, depressed, fearful, or anxious.

✔ WHAT WE CAN DO...

- See your physician if you suspect your spouse is showing signs of dementia.
- Lean on medical professionals for guidance on ways in which you can help your spouse and manage their symptoms.
- Take comfort in knowing most dementias progress slowly. Plenty of memorable times are ahead.

Spousal Caregivers

Even close friends and family members rarely understand the enormous difficulty of caring for a loved one with Alzheimer's. Unless they spend 24/7 with our spouse, they have no idea of the support our loved one requires. From their perspective, they see a boulder in our path when we know we are climbing a mountain. One can be expected to walk over or around a boulder but a life of climbing the face of a mountain is quite a different story.

One reason other people have difficulty understanding our spouses' condition is that our spouses don't outwardly appear ill. Through much of the disease's long course victims can carry on basic conversations, smile, and appear to engage reasonably with others. Alzheimer's doesn't become obvious until late in the disease's course, when our spouse begins to deteriorate physically.

This façade is not only misleading, it's dangerous. It can prevent our spouses from getting the support they may desperately need. Should they be out on their own and become disoriented, they may not know how to ask for help, and other people aren't likely to be aware that they need it.

One of my fears when Marshall was in the early stages was that we'd be in an accident together, that I would be injured and disabled, leaving him to wander through the streets or down hospital corridors. No one would recognize his need for assistance any more than he would realize his own helplessness. He might not even recognize that he was lost. I began carrying a note in my wallet that says: "In the event of an emergency in which I am unable to respond, be aware my husband, Marshall Brodien, who may be with me, has Alzheimer's disease." It then provides emergency contact information. I carry that note to this day.

Our responsibilities to a spouse with Alzheimer's never end. As the disease progresses, so does the required level of care. We must monitor our spouses' feelings and needs. They may not know if they are hot, cold, hungry, or tired. If they are agitated, and unable to tell us why, we have to figure it out. We are detectives, always striving to find the underlying cause of their discomfort. Did they miss a meal? Is there a draft? Is some article of clothing binding? Are they in pain?

We are our spouses' memory. As their past becomes increasingly jumbled, we help them sort it out. Like an external hard drive, we keep tabs on important data such as past health issues, friend and family connections, appointments they must keep...

Their critical decisions about things like healthcare and finances become our responsibility. We are their money manager, nurse, advocate, housekeeper, and personal assistant. This is all in addition to tending to our own needs, other family members, holding down a job, and managing our household.

Through it all, we listen to endless repetition, the same question or statement spoken over and over again. If our spouses repeatedly express their displeasure with something we have done, it feels as if we are continuously being attacked. Until we learn to turn that off, it can be grating. Even with that discipline, it is wearing on the more difficult days.

Responsibilities also become increasingly more physically demanding. There is a lot of lifting, and they may need assistance with walking, bathing, dressing, toileting. And everything in their trail needs to be constantly cleaned as they are messy eaters and bathroom users.

Doctor visits and tests fill our schedule. Medications must be monitored and changes in health have to be addressed. This is one obligation that can't be pushed off.

Gatekeeper is another title we've added to our repertoire as we must guard them and their activities. This is a position we don't want to be in any more than they want us to be in it. They are adults, not children or prisoners, and often chafe at the continuing erosion of personal power. But we protect them for their own good. Their actions are so often irrational.

As gatekeepers, one of the many things we monitor is their careless spending. The concept of money and its value has little meaning to them. We become quite unpopular with outsiders when we stop payment on our spouses' most generous checks.

Their continuous safety is a priority that isn't easily achieved. Keeping a grown man or woman from wandering out the door takes tremendous gentle persuasion. Spouses may be setting out on what in their mind is an important mission, but it is freezing outside, they're in their pajamas, and they will have no idea where they are once they step beyond the front door. Knowing how to redirect their attention, perhaps saying we need their help inside, is an invaluable tool in our growing repertoire of such devices.

They come to feel secure only in our presence and become our shadow. Panic strikes them if we step out of sight. They are constantly underfoot as we move through the house. We are an inseparable couple at this point.

✔ WHAT WE CAN DO...

- Don't let outsiders' critical comments get you down. It's not just that they *don't* understand; they *cannot* understand.
- Try to enjoy your spouse's constant presence. It will be gone someday.
- Ask your spouse to assist you or take over little jobs. They still need to feel valued.

Dealing with the Stress

Surveys repeatedly reveal that Alzheimer's caregivers describe their own stress level as dangerously high. Extreme chronic stress will impair our immunity and corrode our emotional wellbeing. We are at elevated risk of developing cardiovascular disease, impaired kidney function, slow wound healing, hypertension, and stroke.

Recognizing signs of our own stress enables us to take steps to relieve it before our health deteriorates. Sure signs of stress include denial about the disease and its effect on our spouse, anger, social withdrawal, anxiety, depression, exhaustion, sleeplessness, irritability, poor concentration, and an exacerbation of our own pre-existing mental or physical health problems.

30% of caregivers of Alzheimer's disease victims pass away before the person they care for. More shocking is that spousal caregivers in their 60s and older have a 63% higher mortality rate than non-caregivers of the same age.

The strain is severe because of the intensity of care required and the long hours during which we remain under duress. There is no respite for the Alzheimer's spouse. We can't step away. Once it becomes unsafe for our spouse to be left alone, we are together every minute of every day for what may be many years. Our partner needs every last bit of us. The unrelenting onslaught of worry and responsibility often takes us down faster than our spouse.

How we'd love to have someone with whom to discuss *our* difficult day. But the person we most relied on for such support is no longer there. We lost that person when our spouse began to stumble over basic concepts or forget something we said just seconds before. An attempt to speak with them about the struggles we face would only hurt their feelings. Do they really need to understand the burden their condition has placed on us?

We can't talk with our spouse and we can't get away to speak with anyone else. Opportunities to catch up with friends and family members who might offer a sympathetic ear are extremely limited. Little to no time is available to see them or even communicate by email, text, or phone.

Our independence is lost when our loved one can no longer be left alone. We can't get away, and our spouse, diminished as he or she is, has little left to offer us. They need us, every bit of us, always. The isolation and loneliness mount inexorably with each passing day.

Looking at the wide range of devastating symptoms, the unending list of responsibilities that come with them, and the inevitable damage to our own well-being, it's clear why caring for a spouse with Alzheimer's confounds and overwhelms us. The load is impossible for one person to bear alone. A moment of saving grace only comes when we finally understand that although it is our responsibility to ensure these tasks are accomplished, we don't have to, nor can we, do them alone.

✔ WHAT WE CAN DO...

- Practice a relaxation technique like meditation or mindfulness.
- Focus on one task at a time rather than everything that needs to be done. Try to do only what is doable. Let go of what is not.
- Don't worry about what may never happen.

Daily Routine

The first few years after Marshall was diagnosed, he remained fairly independent. He might not have remembered if he had breakfast or be able to find the bathroom in the middle of the night, but he could manage his personal grooming and daily living needs with just a few reminders. He showered, shaved, and toileted without assistance. We worked well as a team and experienced, for a time, a new appreciation of being together.

The challenges mounted as his need for help grew. One of the greatest obstacles in caring for loved ones with Alzheimer's disease is they typically are unable to recognize their limitations. They believe themselves capable of attending to their own needs. In fact, they believe—however much assistance they may require—that they do everything themselves.

We went out to dinner together the evening after Marshall and I received the final results of his neuropsychological test, and the confirmation that he did indeed appear to have Alzheimer's disease. The diagnosis wasn't surprising, but still, it left me stunned. I could barely speak while we sat in our booth in the restaurant. At one point, Marshall stood up to use the restroom. He looked down at me and burst out laughing. Marshall said it was hilarious to see me so sad. That reaction signaled all too clearly to me the difficulties that lay ahead.

At this time, Marshall is in the late stages of Alzheimer's and needs assistance with nearly everything he does. But if you ask him, he will tell you he is fully independent. The thought that he cannot cut up his food or shower without help is unfathomable and insulting to him. He believes he handles all his affairs—drives, pays bills, travels, and entertains crowds regularly—when in fact, everything is done for him. He requires assistance with the most basic daily living activities.

This inability to recognize the need for support is common. People with Alzheimer's can be dependent on a wheelchair for years yet try to walk on their own. They simply forget they can no longer walk.

Overseeing their hygiene also is an essential responsibility to prevent infections. And it is one of the greatest stressors of the day for both the giver and the receiver of care. Our loved one can feel quite vulnerable as we remove their clothes, stand them naked in the shower, and spray them with water. In addition, they're easily chilled, even when the water and room are warm.

Every step must be taken with patience as they move slowly and argumentatively through the day. They are in no hurry, have little energy, and are, after all, still adults. It isn't as if we can pick them up and sit them in the tub like a child. We must calmly persist in coaxing them through the process of caring for them without upsetting or demeaning them.

We can bribe them, though. Offering a reward like ice cream or potato chips after completing an activity they are resisting is usually a good means of getting them to comply.

Several attempts may be necessary before they finally agree to our request. Or they may not cooperate at all. At that point it is best to just let it go. Tomorrow will be another day.

The only issue over which we can't compromise is medication. No matter how much they resist, especially if they need pharmaceutical assistance to eliminate hallucinations or control depression and paranoia, we must insist. These drugs are ineffective if they aren't administered correctly.

✓ WHAT WE CAN DO...

- Cue your spouse with little reminders such as setting out their toothbrush and toothpaste so they remember to brush their teeth.
- Sort pills into weekly organizers to eliminate having to do this daily and to assure a dose is not missed. Some pharmaceutical services will even do this for you.
- Remind yourself that it isn't the end of the world if your spouse does not comply with your non-medical requests.

The Question They're Really Asking

"What can you tell me about Marshall today?" asks my friend, Sue. She's a psychologist and understands that the common question, "How is Marshall?" isn't easy to answer. When I'm asked that question, I respond, "Good, considering." Marshall's certainly not good. He's not healthy. But he is good, considering he has Alzheimer's disease.

Sue's is the better question, and it's really what caring friends are asking. They want to know how our loved one is doing at this moment in time. Are they frightened or hurting emotionally or physically? How does this dementia thing work? What's happening with them right now?

It's also what they want to know about us. They are interested in what we can tell them. After all, they care about us and may be in the same position someday. What we share may be helpful in their future.

And in its wording a question like Sue's permits us to leave out the things we cannot or do not want to tell them.

Answering the question of how we are doing ourselves is often as difficult as talking about a spouse. How rarely do we stop to think about our own needs?

One thing I remind myself of regularly is how grateful I am for the years we had when Marshall was in good health. He was a devoted, loving husband and so very kind to my children. He brought laughter into our home and a joy we'd never experienced before. As challenging as our current life is, I'm honored to care for the man I love, the man who once cared so very much for me.

That vow to endure through sickness and in health is so much more than standing by during a bout of the flu or even a surgery or two. Few of us anticipate that times could ever be as trying as providing years of Alzheimer's care.

The role of long-term caregiver brings with it an unforeseeable abundance of sweat and tears. We never received any formal education to prepare us for this role. We must be self-teachers, trapped on an uncharted path of hands-on self-training and learning from our mistakes. But here we are, giving all we have, giving all we are to our spouses, supporting, caring for, and loving them through their illness as we once vowed we would do.

✔ WHAT WE CAN DO...

- Think beyond the Alzheimer's when asked how your spouse is doing. They are so much more than their disease.
- Enjoy the good moments. There always are some we should not miss.
- Recognize that caring for a spouse in their greatest time of need is in one sense a privilege, not just a gift we give but one we receive, the privilege of being able to offer ourselves to them in a way no one else ever can.

Communicating with Alzheimer's

No marriage really works well for both partners without good communication. As spouses, we share our thoughts, worries, and aspirations. We work out our problems in our relationship and confront together the most difficult issues in life. We use each other as sounding boards and voices of reason. We mentor, console, and inspire one another.

Effective communication depends on each party respecting what the other has to say, listening attentively, and acknowledging our understanding of what was said. Constructive criticism and advice can be offered because each partner is equally heard and understood, or at least believes an honest attempt to understand has been made. We grow not just individually through such interactions, but as a couple. We empower one another and strengthen the bonds of our union.

The failure of good communication is another consequence of Alzheimer's. As the disease progresses, the spouse with mid-to-late Alzheimer's cannot follow what the other says—ever. They don't remember words spoken only moments ago. The message received is often jumbled and twisted. A single word or phrase may be misunderstood and latched on to, resulting in an argument that can go nowhere useful.

Marshall and I had countless attempts at a discussion during the early part of this disease when he seemed only to hear one word I had spoken and fixated on it. He was certain I had said something hurtful and there was no way to convince him otherwise or redirect his mounting anger. The only alternative to ending his rant was to let him go on about words I had never spoken without commenting further. Sometimes you just have to stop putting fuel on the fire.

So much of the communication between couples with Alzheimer's is counter to traditional conversation. The disease requires us to react in a most unnatural way. It is normal to challenge a spouse who says something ridiculous. It is normal to defend ourselves when accused of something we did not say, or some hurtful thing we would never do.

Neither challenging what they say nor defending ourselves is helpful when Alzheimer's is involved. To do so only fuels a pointless argument. The number one rule in dealing with people with Alzheimer's is: Do not argue with them. You can't reason with someone who no longer has a sense of reason. Explanations or definitions are useless and may only serve to incite their fury.

Rather, we must hold back our own feelings. We swallow our pride and our pain, which is ultimately unhealthy for us, but it is the only way to allow the "discussion" to resolve itself. As much as it bridles, we allow our spouses to express their anger without an opportunity to express our own.

Nor can we always tell the truth. Lies are essential in preventing our spouse from enduring unnecessary distress. If the thought of an upcoming doctor appointment upsets them, we don't tell them about it. We leave the house with them and say we are going shopping. If we know that a long day out with friends is too much for them, and they insistent on going, we tell them it has been canceled. When we go for a haircut and a friend stays with our spouse because our spouse cannot be left alone, we say the friend just wanted to visit.

Our marital conversations test our own sanity as nothing has before. How often Marshall has told me that I am crazy. What I am saying is so strange to him. He finds me odd. Ironically, I must admit there have been countless times when our conversations went in such an irrational direction that I wondered if he might not be right. I was so confused at the end of some attempts at conversation that I had no idea where we started or how we ended up where we did.

✔ WHAT WE CAN DO...

- Don't argue. Disagreeing with your spouse will only frustrate both of you.
- Tell your spouse what is easiest for them to accept even if it isn't true.
- Avoid long explanations. Keep your conversations short, direct, and calm.

Listening from the Heart

Most of us have a tendency to fix things, to jump in and try to make things right. With Alzheimer's, we can't always do that. We can't correct our spouses' misunderstanding or convince them they're wrong. On the other hand, we don't need to agree with what they are saying either.

What our spouses want is to be heard and understood. Listening without contradicting or judging, no matter how peculiar what they are saying is, will ease their frustration. By looking at them sincerely, listening attentively, and placing a gentle hand on theirs, we can help them to calm down and help restore harmony to the house.

This is the perfect occasion to remember a phrase from the prayer traditionally attributed to St. Francis of Assisi, "Grant that

I may not seek so much to be consoled as to console; to be understood as to understand; to be loved as to love."

What our spouses need most is to be consoled, understood, and loved unconditionally. This is true regardless of the fact that they cannot offer such support in return.

Caring for a loved one with Alzheimer's requires us to act selflessly. No matter how painful, we must put our own feelings aside. We can deal with our emotions at a later date, perhaps with friends, a counselor, or clergy.

Our own attitude is often reflected in the behavior of our loved one. When we are tense, they get tense. If we are agitated, they will increasingly become so too. They pick up on our behavior and reflect it. If we want our spouse to remain calm, we need to model serenity for them.

No matter how hurtful, insensitive, or shocking their behavior may be to us, it's best to allow them to express themselves freely. They aren't likely to sense our feelings or understand that they are speaking or acting in a hurtful way. They can be quite detached emotionally. In later stages, even informing them of the death of a close family member will not prompt a reaction of sadness.

Delusions, any firmly held belief in things that are not real, and paranoia are other common symptoms that may appear in mid-to-late stages of Alzheimer's disease. Hallucinations, false perceptions of objects or events that are sensory in nature, also may occur. Trying to convince spouses that their worries are unfounded will only agitate them further. They believe something disturbing truly happened, and if we argue they interpret our behavior as insensitivity to their legitimate fears.

Here is when it is best for us to listen closely and say little or nothing in response. When able, we can redirect their attention to something less upsetting. Surprisingly, they may not even remember their moment of terror a few minutes later.

Non-judgmental listening and avoiding arguments that can have no positive result will prompt a new, better, conversation. Although such talks may be one-sided, we can converse with them as long as they have the power to formulate words. They may express themselves with a limited vocabulary, often with a heavy dose of incorrect word usage. By listening patiently, we offer them the opportunity to feel safe in expressing themselves to us.

I'm surprised at how often I know what Marshall is trying to tell me even when the words he uses make no sense. Our history together allows me to read between the lines, to understand the emotion behind the jumbled words he is using to express himself. And he takes comfort in knowing I have heard him.

This is particularly important to keep in mind when our spouse is showing signs of distress. They may be very obviously angry, but the source of their anger may not be what they are talking about. Their words often do not align with their actions.

A wife may tell her husband she hates him and is leaving him forever when what she really is trying to say is that she doesn't want to eat her broccoli. She might not even recognize what it is that is upsetting. We have to listen with our hearts if we want to understand them more clearly.

✔ WHAT WE CAN DO...

- Listen attentively. It takes tremendous energy for your spouse to express themselves.
- Avoid responding to everything your spouse says, particularly things that may irritate you.
- Try to understand what your spouse is trying to say when what they are actually saying is unintelligible or incoherent.

Deafening Silence

The flip side of incomprehensible conversation is the lack of any conversation at all. As the disease progresses, language skills diminish, and may eventually disappear altogether. Initially, we may witness our loved ones having difficulty finding the right word. They can repeat themselves a shocking number of times. Language skills progressively lessen over time until many Alzheimer's sufferers say nothing at all.

This makes dinner conversation strained to say the least. If you have never dined with someone who looks intently down at their food through an entire meal you can only imagine how uncomfortable that can be. You may ramble on about your day, about news from family or friends, and not get a twinge of response. We are with our spouses 24/7, but they are not really with us in any meaningful way.

One thing Marshall and I often could discuss was food. Our conversation, as far as one could call it that, might go something like this:

"Do you like your dinner?"
"What dinner?"
"Do you like your lasagna?"
"What's that?"
"The food you are eating? Do you like it?"
"I like it. Is this soup?"
"No, Marshall, it's lasagna."
"Ok, I'll go there."

Imagine multiplying that conversation three times each day, day after day, year after year, and you will begin to understand how one can feel lonelier at the table with your spouse than when dining alone.

✔ WHAT WE CAN DO...

- Speak about what's on your mind regardless of whether or not they respond. Your spouse may just enjoy the sound of your voice.
- Play soft music while eating to create a relaxing atmosphere.
- Ask simple questions. Not "What would you like for dinner?" but "Would you like cheese on your hamburger?"

Remembering Our History

One of the saddest losses after years of marriage is being unable to reminisce together. Alzheimer's is a thief. It hijacks our loved ones and steals our most precious memories, the memories that bind us as spousal partners.

Marshall remembers who I am but can recall nothing of our decades of marriage. I cannot talk with him about our past. We can't reminisce about our many good times, travels, family milestones, favorite holidays, or the magic shows we took such joy in working on together. Conversations about the fun we had with friends or the warm glow of special family celebrations are nonexistent. Memories of our life together have vanished as magically as any rabbit in a magician's hat.

Alzheimer's causes its initial damage in the hippocampus, the part of the brain that forms new memories. As neurons die, the brain begins to shrink. This shrinking continues across the brain, progressively claiming old memories as well. The progressive destruction of brain tissue makes it increasingly difficult to form new memories and damages the pathways we must follow to retrieve old ones.

During less advanced stages of their disease, we can reminisce with them and prompt memories, perhaps by peering through old photo albums or watching old home videos. The risk is that doing so can excite feelings of melancholy, for us as well as for them. Some small detail may spark a memory, even if it is only fleeting. Remembering how good life used to be, and can never be again, is painful.

Also painful is recognizing that they cannot identify loved ones in those photos. We surround them with pictures to remind them of all those dear to us, only to hear our spouses ask who all those people are and why their pictures are in our house. In late stages, some Alzheimer's patients may not even be able to recognize their own image.

Because he was a television celebrity, there are many video clips of Marshall on YouTube. Periodically, a friend will send a link to one that particularly touches them, and I'm always surprised at the mix of emotions they stir in me. I love seeing Marshall entertaining, vibrant, and happy. But realizing the man in the video is gone forever is a knife in the heart.

We caregivers are the memory-keepers in the marriage. Memories of those cherished times now are for our benefit only. Alzheimer's wiped them from our spouses' mind, but not ours. We hold them close to our heart to remind us that all those wonderful times we shared were real. We were blessed to have had such occasions as a couple.

Barbara and Bill have been married almost fifty years. According to Bill, they had a nearly perfect marriage until the last few years when dementia crept in. He is angry that after all those beautiful times together their joyful relationship must end in sadness and tears. His energetic, witty wife is completely dependent on him and her other caregivers. Their once lengthy discussions are reduced to a spattering of incoherent words. Barbara now clings to Bill and is openly fearful of the world around her.

The proportion of healthy years to those of illness will differ for each couple, but the pain remains the same. Most of my marriage to Marshall has included Alzheimer's. The majority of Barbara and Bill's has not. We are equally angry that Alzheimer's destroyed our happy marriages.

No matter how long we are married, or what percentage of our marriage is consumed with this disease, we can't help but ask why this happened to us. Why did we have to lose the ability to communicate with our partner, the one we shared our sorrows and joys with? Our spouse is still with us, but his or her ability to help us sail through life is gone.

So much of Alzheimer's is so very disturbing that it is all too easy to overlook what we have had, and what we do still have. As long as our spouses are alive, they are present to us in some way. Something of them, and of us as a couple, remains until one of us takes a last breath.

Marshall still tells me he loves me and that I am the love of his life. Although, he doesn't say these things as often as he used to, I cherish hearing those words every time he utters them. I pray they are the last ones I hear from him.

✔ WHAT WE CAN DO...

- Peer through old photos recalling favorite shared events and people close to you.
- Pack away mementos too painful to revisit right now. Recognize that you're very likely to appreciate them again someday.
- Continue to create new memories with your spouse.

Alzheimer's at Home

Marriage revolves around home and family. We get married and we nest. We build a family that may be comprised in any variety of ways. Whether it's traditional mother, father and kids, a blended group of children from prior marriages, or just an assortment of furry creatures, our great dream is to build a safe haven for all our loves.

When a member of our family is unable to continue in their established role, the overall dynamic of the family changes. All members of the family feel the loss when one cannot carry on as their typical self. The old center does not hold. The whole family must make major adjustments.

With the intrusion of Alzheimer's, Mom, Dad, or a sibling is still alive, and physically well, but their role is significantly diminished due to their cognitive limitations. And their decline is progressive; we no sooner adjust to a new normal than we are confronted by another downward slip.

We grieve all along the Alzheimer's trail of destruction. Something new is always prompting us to mourn. Memories vanish. Our loved one becomes emotionally detached. Their absence at family gatherings is a sore reminder of their present state. Everything we cherish is lost little by little.

No matter how well we manage to come to terms with what is happening, it's still painful. My brother-in-law tells of a dinner when he and his two brothers sat at the table with his parents. His mother, who was well into Alzheimer's at the time, remarked how much the three men looked alike. "Are you related?" she asked. They chuckled, but how could they not also feel a pang of sorrow at how removed their mother had become from her own children?

And the disease can bring down the primary caregiver just as ruthlessly as it brings down the spouse with Alzheimer's. That means us. The impact of the disease on the primary caregiver is so devastating that we are commonly referred to as a second victim of the disease. We experience a poorer quality of life, a higher susceptibility to serious illness, social isolation, anger, guilt, emotional distress—often including depression—and financial hardship. The family stands in jeopardy of losing two members as a direct result of the disease's assault on one of us. At the very least, the family loses some of both of us all along the way as the time we have left to meet their needs shrinks month by month.

Marshall and I have a blended family. When we married, we brought together his four children, aged eighteen to thirty-one, and my three, aged thirteen through nineteen. Each one has a special relationship with Marshall, and of course we all love him very much. Watching his decline has been agonizing in a different way for each of us.

I'm especially saddened for my step-children. It's painful to see that their father recognizes their faces as familiar but doesn't know them as his children. He doesn't remember their names or any of their happy times together. His memories of holding them, playing with them—even loving them—are gone.

My step-children mourn the loss of a shared joy in childhood memories, but just as poignantly the loss of an adult relationship with their father, one they always expected they would have but do not enjoy today. They can't go to their father for guidance, as so many of us do. In addition to missing that fatherly direction and love, the evidence that Alzheimer's is inheritable weighs heavily on them.

That is a cause for concern that most families share. The source of this fear is the fact that researchers aren't entirely certain why the risk of developing the disease is higher in some families. Genetic testing can offer some indication of risk, but a positive result does not tell us definitely that we will develop it, and a negative result is no guarantee that we will not. The decision to take the test at all is a very personal one, with no assurance one way or the other of whether and when Alzheimer's may develop.

We all begin our trek through this experience understanding that our loved one's memory will continue to fade. We know that they will progressively forget people close to them. But we are never prepared for the day that forgotten person turns out to be us. We can't help but cling to the desperate hope that we are too special to be forgotten, even though we know on an intellectual level that "special" has nothing to do with it.

✓ WHAT WE CAN DO...

- Discuss your feelings about Alzheimer's candidly with the rest of your family.
- Investigate the risk factors of Alzheimer's specific to your family.
- Be tolerant of each family member's method of processing your loved one's illness. Others may not handle difficulties the same way you do.

Talk it Out

The effect of Alzheimer's on individual family members will often drive interactions throughout the family. The reality that one of us has Alzheimer's ripples out among our close relatives, triggering an often-vast range of emotions. Anger, fear, frustration, jealousy, guilt, and sadness can easily provoke conflicts among family members struggling to deal with a loved one's slow but inevitable decline.

Sandra enjoyed a close relationship with her mother but felt her father, who was much older, often stood between them. She always assumed her father would pass away first and, when he did, she and her mother would spend more quality time together. But her mother's recent diagnosis of Alzheimer's has made her realize those days will never come. The twist of fate is disturbing and disappointing for her. She is experiencing a mix of anger and guilt.

Having a spouse with Alzheimer's puts our relationships with other family members under considerable stress. Caring for our spouse consumes so much of our time that we have little left for anyone else. Because we are so involved in caring for our spouse, we tend to lose touch with more distant family members and lose precious time with our children and grandchildren. The disappointment we suffer over lost opportunities with them and the diminishing chances to find moments of family joy can engender feelings of resentment and frustration.

Families of a person experiencing early-onset dementia face extraordinary challenges in just keeping themselves afloat. Many of these families include teen-agers or young children who will miss out on valuable time spent with their healthy parent as well as their sick one. As the parent with Alzheimer's progressively needs more care, the healthy one will have less and less time for the children.

A parent with Alzheimer's may unknowingly mistreat their children. They may cause them life-long emotional—even physical—harm. Many people with Alzheimer's drive with their children in the car, use power tools, and cook without supervision long after they should have stopped. How easily, and unthinkingly, they can put their children and other loved ones in danger.

Teenage children often become resentful or feel embarrassed about their ill parent, with consequent feelings of anger and guilt that can disrupt the whole family. These adolescents are not likely to have peers with the emotional depth necessary to console them. Their friends have probably not yet known anyone with dementia. It's important to call in professional help for these children as early as possible. The guidance of a well-trained and sympathetic school social worker can assist them enormously in dealing with their burgeoning negative emotions.

There is much to sort through emotionally when Alzheimer's strikes the family. It's highly beneficial to encourage children of all ages to talk about their feelings. Gentle, compassionate conversations about what each person in the family is feeling throughout the disease can not only ease each member's pain but the group's shared suffering as well. A united family can better remember its past and mourn together, in sympathetic harmony, the losses they endure.

✔ **WHAT WE CAN DO...**

- Enroll children in counseling to offer them a completely nonjudgmental person with whom they can express their feelings. Don't wait for signs of distress.
- Forgive yourself, and others, for past shortcomings and move forward with love and compassion.
- Know that the continuous losses due to Alzheimer's require continuous adjustment in your own understanding and mourning.

Working as a Team

Alzheimer's offers families countless opportunities to work together. Responsibilities need to be shared to prevent one member from burning out completely. Such team work actually serves to strengthen the family as a whole.

I saw this hidden blessing with my parents and siblings when my parents were ill. Although my parents suffered with cancer and not dementia, there was a lot to be done, and my siblings and I divided responsibilities and worked very well together. We assumed responsibilities according to our capabilities, overseeing doctor appointments and medications, assisting with meals and housecleaning, making the endless necessary phone calls, managing the lawn care and snow removal, and handling all the financial concerns. Since my parents' deaths, we continue to share a special bond strengthened by the adversity we faced together.

Unfortunately, few families manage to distribute the load equally and hard feelings often ensue. The vast majority of emails I receive are from family members who complain that their siblings or children do not help as much as needed. One member typically carries the bulk of the load while the others pop in from time to time.

There are many reasons for the lack of teamwork. A family may be spread out across the country with some members having to endure long travel times and significant expense to visit. An individual family member may be overloaded with career responsibilities and the needs of their immediate family. Petty jealousies arise; personalities collide. Understandable disagreements about how things should be done can always be a hindrance to unified action. Some family members just feel unqualified or emotionally unable to help.

And if our spouse was previously married, it can be even more challenging. Typically, step-children are less helpful. Their focus tends to remain on their parent, and they aren't as concerned about the step-parent. They are less aware of how they can assist their step-parent in caring for their birth parent or how difficult the situation truly is. As long as their birth parent is cared for, they don't feel the particular need to volunteer any assistance.

The ones who do jump in find themselves locked in emotionally charged experiences that can be both heartwarming and heartaching. These encounters give them some final opportunities to create new memories that they can hold on to and treasure long after their loved one is gone. And we can find a supreme feeling of satisfaction in knowing we were involved in doing something vital to the well being of our whole family.

Anna and Joel cared for three of their parents living in their home, all three with different forms of dementia, while their two children were still teenagers. The household was lively, to say the least. Each grandparent needed different kinds of attention. As trying as that time may have been, it offered their children important life lessons, some not so easily come by. They learned what a family is all about and how each member accepts responsibility for every other. Their exposure to aging and illness offered them opportunities to learn about compassion and how to address the demanding physical needs of aging adults no longer able to care for themselves. They also shared loving, sweet moments they wouldn't have had if their grandparents were not in their home, under their care.

When my nephew, Jaymes, was in his mid-twenties, he moved in with his grandparents. His grandmother was in poor health and his grandfather's Alzheimer's was quite advanced. Jaymes took charge of many of his grandfather's daily personal needs, like showering and shaving him, and his grandmother recalls that he offered her steady comedic relief. His quick wit and easy-going personality lightened the dark mood in the house immeasurably. Although emotionally draining, it was a powerful experience that undoubtedly will inspire Jaymes for the rest of his life.

✔ WHAT WE CAN DO...

- Graciously accept the assistance of willing family members. Your loved one is their loved one too.
- Encourage cooperation and division of care, perhaps choosing one family member to oversee insurance claims, another to accompany you and your spouse to the doctors, and others to prepare a few hot meals each week.
- Forgive those who do not offer help. Focus your attention on more important matters.

Alzheimer's Decor

Decorating our shared space is one of the great pleasures (and often great compromises) of making a life together. With a little unavoidable give and take, we meld our different personalities and varying tastes to create an environment that expresses our new identity as a couple.

When serious illness enters the home, it never fails to make its presence known. Medicine bottles, handlebars, oxygen tanks, walkers, and wheel chairs are suddenly scattered through the house. Along with the progressive decline in health comes a parade of medical devices, locks, and alarms. The home becomes more functional and secure, and less beautiful, and a new aesthetic emerges to serve a higher imperative: the safety and comfort of a seriously incapacitated person.

Stairways and steps may need to be gated to prevent our spouse from using them without assistance. Alzheimer's can interfere with depth perception, so even small steps and irregularities in flooring pose tripping hazards, with considerable risk of injury. Our bones become brittle with age and can fracture and break with the impact of even a minor fall.

Area rugs and runners will need to be removed. Even bathroom mats under sinks can be dangerous. If we want to use them while we are at the sink, we may need to put them down temporarily and then pick them up when we are finished.

Since we must now spend so many hours offering care, keeping the home decor simple is also helpful in reducing time-consuming chores. Fewer knick knacks lessen the need to dust. Keeping the daily menu simple reduces time in the kitchen.

I tend to complicate things more than I need to. I love to cook from scratch and have always prided myself on keeping an immaculate house. Neither of these goals is realistic when we are already pushed to our limits, and we have to find it in ourselves to let them go. Caring for our loved one dominates so much of our time that what remains needs to be prudently rationed.

Wandering is another common consequence of Alzheimer's. Our spouse may think they have an important engagement or want to go to work. But once out the door they can become very disoriented. The neighborhood they once loved to stroll through is now unrecognizable to them. If wandering grows to be a regular issue, it may be wise to install a security system with alarms on the doors to signal when someone slips out.

Potential hazards loom everywhere: inside, outside, and all around the house. Some dangers aren't apparent until after an accident. We have to search our homes thoroughly and secure all sharp items or chemicals that might prove dangerous: kitchen knives, screwdrivers, utility and hobby knives, razors, garden tools, snips, scissors, kitchen utensils, fragile glass objects, cleaning supplies, small engine fuel and oil, paint thinner, lubricants, prescriptions, propane tanks, matches, lighters…you may even need to install stove safety knobs or cut-offs for the fuel supply to your kitchen range.

Power tools, saws, and even lawn mowers that once were commonly used by our loved ones now pose serious safety risks. Our spouses may have been quite handy—an expert gardener, perhaps, or the neighborhood's go-to automotive mechanic—but things have changed. They no longer can remember how to complete even a simple task and the tools they once used safely can cause them serious harm.

We no more want to take these activities, tools, and sources of pleasure from our spouse than they want them removed. And most likely, they won't understand why we must. They don't realize they can no longer safely handle these once-familiar tools. As we learn so soon, most people with Alzheimer's disease are oblivious to their decline. For their own safety we have to sneak these items out of the house or secure them when our spouse is not around.

Marshall owned several magic tricks that posed a potential risk. One consisted of three wooden disks, one of which had a long spike sticking up through the middle of it. The trick begins with the magician covering each disk with a common Styrofoam coffee cup, perhaps borrowed from the audience or pulled at random from a newly opened package. The magician then turns around while a spectator rearranges the three cups to his satisfaction. The magician turns and quickly crushes two of the cups with two quick blows of his flattened hand and, with a practiced flourish, to a round of astonished applause, lifts the third cup to reveal the long spike.

A good magician is always certain beyond a doubt which cup hides the spike (of course I will not reveal how!) and is never at the slightest risk of injury. But as talented as Marshall once had been, his powers of observation and his memory both diminished with the disease, and there came a time when he could no longer perform the trick safely. After I watched him strike his hand against a spike during one performance, the disks themselves magically disappeared. He looked everywhere but couldn't seem to recall where he had put them. I was relieved when he soon forgot the trick was ever part of his repertoire.

✔ WHAT WE CAN DO...

- Secure exits with locks and alarms to prevent wandering.
- Install safety latches on medicine cabinets and any doors or drawers that enclose anything potentially dangerous.
- Rid the home and garage of candles, lighters, power tools, and other objects that may present a hazard.

Our Home Museum

Marshall reveled in an exciting life of celebrity that included stints as a side-show talker at carnivals, a practicing professional magician, MC for an ice show, trade show entertainer, TV personality Wizzo the Wizard on Chicago's Bozo Show, and creator of TV Magic Cards. Our 1,000-square foot basement game room was transformed into an extensive museum featuring highlights of Marshall's career-newspaper clippings, costumes, and artifacts.

As the years passed in our lovely, spacious home, it became increasingly evident that we needed to downsize. The home was too expensive and required too much maintenance. The only work that Marshall was doing were volunteer and guest appearances, and my time available to work gainfully was shrinking as his need for care grew. His Alzheimer's required my attention night and day.

I knew that moving would have many drawbacks—not the least of which would be closing the museum. It gave Marshall a sense of purpose. He spent endless hours down there moving things around and peering through photo albums. He invited guests—all the time—to see it. And they came. Visitors showed up at the door without my expecting them or Marshall even remembering that he had invited them. Once they entered the homage we had built to his long and happy career, everyone laughed, oohed and aahed, and Marshall's lifelong drive to entertain others was fulfilled once more.

But two of the symptoms of Alzheimer's disease are paranoia and delusions. These symptoms became more evident with every guest. The moment a visitor was gone, Marshall would report to me his suspicion that they had stolen something, or claim they had somehow acted inappropriately, or was convinced he had done something inappropriate himself.

An activity that had once kept him busy and offered me a welcome break to complete some neglected chores now required my monitoring presence. As each guest arrived, I had to follow them and Marshall through the museum. I'm sure many thought I was intrusive, but it was necessary for everyone's well-being, not least of all Marshall's. I finally began to discourage acquaintances from visiting to avoid the risk to Marshall's reputation.

So, the museum posed a difficult dilemma. If we moved to a smaller home, Marshall would be left in front of the television when I could not entertain him. If we stayed, the house would continue to devour time and money now needed elsewhere. I had no choice but to leave things as they were until Marshall was moved into assisted living for memory care. It was only then that I was able to disassemble the museum and ready the house for sale.

✔ WHAT WE CAN DO...

- Declutter as much as you can as often as you can.
- Avoid removing your spouse's favorite items when he or she is around.
- Keep stairways and doorways free of clutter.

Home Sweet Home

Our home is our haven. It's where we go to shut out the rest of the world, for peace and quiet. But as our spouses require an ever-increasing level of care, we may need to call in assistance. Other family members may have to cover for us so we can attend to our personal needs or get some important respite. If family members are unwilling or unable to step up, hiring caregivers must be given serious consideration.

The extra help lightens our burdens. Our spouses may be more compliant with strangers than they are with us. And they will ultimately be far safer with another set of eyes watching out for them. We also gain companionship ourselves. Assistants offer us someone to talk to and consult with, someone to empathize with and console us.

That is not to say there aren't any drawbacks to inviting hired caregivers into the home. When we share caregiving responsibility, we give up a lot of our privacy. We have outsiders coming and going, even living in our homes along with us, and caring for our spouse in their own way. We lose control of both home and spouse.

All the disruption in comfortable routines may also cause our spouses to become agitated. They know things aren't normal and are stressed by that fact. We can be affected emotionally ourselves because of this invasive new normal. Our house no longer feels like home to either one of us.

Toward the end of the time Marshall was at home, I became seriously ill and required bed rest. The doctor insisted on our hiring additional caregivers to care for Marshall, especially at night, until I recovered.

Since no caregiver works 24/7 as we spouses must, multiple aides worked in shifts. Marshall disliked the resulting rotation. He wanted things to be like they had been before, without even fully remembering how that was.

The last year or so Marshall lived in our house, the house we shared for nearly twenty years, he'd ask repeatedly, "When are we going home?" It took me a while to understand that he had forgotten his own home while still living in it. He often couldn't find the bathroom or figure out how to get upstairs or down.

Marshall's muddled version of home is a place that does not exist in reality. He imagines a combination of several homes he lived in, mostly during his childhood and younger years. This "home" he insists on going back to is somewhere I am powerless to take him.

And now that he lives in a memory care community, he, like many residents living in such places, periodically asks again when he can go home. The question is disturbing even though I understand that it is not our house he is longing for. Knowing that there will never be a place where he can fully feel at home again saddens me so deeply.

I comfort Marshall by reminding him that he is surrounded by his belongings. I point out his photos, clothes, and shoes. As his level of security has progressively grown in his present home, he has become increasingly uneasy outside the safety of that door.

What he's really looking for is me. I'm home. He is most comfortable retreating into his memory community—with me—until he forgets me too.

✔ WHAT WE CAN DO...

- Call in caregivers early in the disease so they become part of the daily routine.
- Understand there will be things your spouse longs for that no one, not even you, can provide for them.
- Designate a part of your house as your sanctuary, your own private space, when caregivers are working in your home.

Date Night with Alzheimer's

Marriage allows us to date our favorite person for the rest of our lives—dinner, movies, plays, sporting events, and parties enjoyed with the person we love most in the world. Whether dressed to the nines in a five-star restaurant or snuggled on the couch in our jammies, we get to play together for the remainder of our days. And many couples do enjoy a happy and fulfilling marriage for many decades.

But date night takes on a whole new meaning when Alzheimer's tags along. We may celebrate Valentine's Day in a romantic restaurant not only ordering a meal for our spouse but cutting up their food. We have to guess at what they might be in the mood for tonight and if they will be able to manage eating it. We can't go by what they may have preferred in the past. And if they need to use the restroom, the outing can quickly take a downward spiral, even a messy one.

Peter and Marion's 50th wedding anniversary is fast approaching. Peter recognizes that their golden anniversary will not be the celebratory event he once envisioned it would be. They won't dine out with family in a nice restaurant as hoped. Marion recently moved into memory care. The restaurant setting would be too upsetting for her. Peter, in all honesty, prefers not to put her eating habits on public display. He feels a need to protect her dignity.

Everything changes with Alzheimer's. As the disease progresses, people with the disease can forget their dining preferences. Their ability to cut, chew, and swallow is compromised. The lively restaurant setting they once enjoyed may now be intrusive and disturbing. Any hearing deficit—a common accompanying condition—will make it difficult for them to understand us from across the table in a noisy room.

We shouldn't be surprised if our spouses keep their head down toward their food the entire meal. They are submerged in the depths of sensory overload, unable to separate our words from the scrape of chairs, the murmur of other conversations, and the clink of dinnerware. The stress of striving to remain focused amidst so much distraction can easily cause them to shut down.

All that was once familiar grows progressively unfamiliar to our spouses. The comforts of a favorite restaurant can no longer be anticipated with pleasure and the friendly wait staff that has always welcomed us are now strangers to them. And after our best efforts for a lovely dinner together, we walk out the door, leftovers still in hand, as our loved ones ask, "Are we going out to eat?"

✔ WHAT WE CAN DO...

- Choose quiet, smaller restaurants or ones divided into small rooms.
- Face your spouse toward a wall in restaurants to reduce distractions.
- Dine with another couple for added assistance and conversation.

Dates for All Stages

We can do a great deal with our spouse throughout most of the disease if we plan carefully and keep an open mind. Depending on the stage our spouse is in, seeking outside entertainment can be more stressful than fun. Finding the appropriate level of activity is the secret to a pleasurable outing for both of us.

Most activities enjoyed before the disease's onset remain doable in the early-to-mid-stages of Alzheimer's. It is better if the activities are planned so they don't exceed our spouses' limit of energy, aren't among large crowds, or don't occur late in the day. Successful dates get trickier over time as our spouses grow more physically and mentally challenged.

Every stimulant consumes our spouses' energy—lights, sounds, smells, movement, and crowds. The greater the total stimulation, the more exhausting the outing will be for them and the more difficult it will be to care for them that evening and even the following day.

The success of these dates varies greatly, depending on how advanced our spouses' Alzheimer's disease is and whether they have any other health issues. We need to be prepared to administer medications, observe diet restrictions, and possibly change their underwear and clothes. Their safety getting in and out of vehicles and walking on unsteady pavement also requires careful planning and execution.

Since Alzheimer's rapidly drains our spouses' energy, they will prefer smaller groups than they did in the past. The fewer people around them, the less stress they'll experience. If their traditional preference was to socialize in intimate groups, large crowds are likely to upset them even further.

Their choice of movies and television shows will change along the way. When they can no longer track the plot as the story unfolds, dramas will become rather boring. Action movies will be entertaining until the point where their intensity becomes overwhelming. Variety and game shows offer a better alternative because they can be easily enjoyed in the moment.

Assisting spouses in and out of the car is another difficulty for both them and us, especially if our own balance is somewhat unstable. We'll need to be able to brace them as they step unsteadily off the curb or their poor depth perception can send us both tumbling to the ground. And then we'll need to cautiously ease them into the seat, lift their legs into the car, and buckle them in.

The following check-list is helpful to run through before venturing out.

Consider:

- The accessibility to our choice of destination. Are there stairs to climb? How steady is the pavement?

- What is the noise level? Is there a quiet corner in the restaurant or a noisy area best avoided?

- How is the lighting? Brighter is usually better.

- Will you be able to assist your spouse in the restroom? If they are incontinent, can you change them there?

- Are you physically strong enough to assist them in and out of a chair and the car?

- If the drive is long, where will you be able to stop along the way if necessary?

And keep in mind that the strain of the outing begins from the time we leave home. If it takes an hour to get where we want to go, our spouse has already expended an hour of energy before the event begins. Because the total time away from familiar surroundings should not exceed two or three hours, we have less than an hour to stay before we must be on our way home.

In the first few years that Marshall showed symptoms of Alzheimer's, we walked nearly every day. We were both in great physical shape and he usually remained emotionally calm. The walk provided us fresh air, sunshine, physical activity, and a daily opportunity to talk about what we saw along the way. We often strolled to a nearby restaurant for lunch before heading back home. I have fond memories of those wonderful times we shared.

Now that Marshall has entered the late stages of the disease, he is no longer able to take long walks. He tires easily and is hunched and unsteady in his gait. Every curb and irregularity in the pavement poses a hazard as he shuffles and struggles to pick up his feet. Although our strolls may take a long time, we cover very little ground.

Our entertainment dates are nonexistent at this point. Magic was his life, but by mid-stage, attending these magic shows began to raise his anxiety level tremendously. He was increasingly more confused about what was happening, who we were with, and what he thought he should be doing. He worried that he was supposed to be working but couldn't remember what to do.

Sadly, he has little interest in these shows anymore. When old friends came to entertain residents at his memory care community, Marshall fell asleep. A trick now and then by his son or close peers is as much magic as he can enjoy.

What works for us now depends on a combination of good luck and careful planning. I must admit that any dates we have shared in recent years were more for me than him. Marshall is just as content staying in his home. Taking a meal outside his room is as much variety as he wants in his life right now.

✔ WHAT WE CAN DO...

- Take little walks in malls or other places with solid footing and good lighting.
- Venture out for a snack or ice cream rather than a full meal.
- Accept that plans may need to be altered or canceled at the last minute.

Identification and Tracking Devices

Once out the door, we have to consider the possibility that we may lose track of our spouses. While we concentrate on which potatoes to buy in the grocery store, or stop for a quick run into the restroom, they may wander out of sight. Most likely, they haven't gone far, and we find them within minutes, but those minutes will be the most stressful of the day.

For our own peace of mind, and for their safety, we have a few options to help track them, or at least identify them should they wander too far off. None are full-proof. Our spouses must cooperate in using them. But the precautions offer some protection once they are in place.

Getting them to carry a cell phone allows us to track them with apps like Find My Friends—as long as they don't lose the phone. The phone is of no value if left in the bathroom or charging on the kitchen counter. They also need to be able to hear the ring or understand that the vibration is signaling them to answer the phone.

Attach an "I HAVE A CONDITION" card next to your spouse's photo ID, and both of you should carry a simple description of your spouse's condition that also provides emergency contact information.

If our spouse will wear one, an ID bracelet offers first responders the best hope of identifying our spouse and contacting us. A variety of bracelets are available from multiple sources, including Amazon and the Alzheimer's Association. MedicAlert® + Alzheimer's Association Safe Return® is a 24-hour nationwide emergency response service. If our spouse wanders off, we can activate a whole community of support with a phone call or two. When he or she is found, first responders will call the number on the bracelet and assist in a safe return. This essential service is eminently affordable, with a modest initial cost for a bracelet and a low annual fee.

✔ WHAT WE CAN DO...

- Persuade a friend to join the two of you on an outing if you expect you may need to be separated from your spouse, even for a short time, for instance taking a restroom break or trying on apparel.
- Inform wait staff and store clerks that your spouse has Alzheimer's if you need to step into a restroom or dressing room.
- Alert local law enforcement of your spouse's condition.
- Ask neighbors to call you immediately if they see your spouse on the street.

Venturing Out of Town

All of these precautions are particularly important when traveling out of town. In addition, a day of rest after traveling in each direction, periodic daily rest periods throughout the vacation, and an early bedtime should all be scheduled into the itinerary.

If flying, alert TSA agents of your spouse's condition before preceding through airport security and notify a flight attendant once on board. This needs to be done as discretely as possible to avoid embarrassing or upsetting your spouse.

You also want to pack smart and travel light so that you have just the necessities, without a lot of extraneous items. Essentials include medications, snacks, emergency contacts, photocopies of important legal documents, medical power of attorney, and insurance cards. If your spouse has sundowners, a condition that makes them increasingly more confused as the day goes on, activities are best planned early in the day. By mid-to-late afternoon, your spouse can become very confused, resulting in a disconcerting outing for both of you. Alzheimer's patients are already disoriented by being thrust into unfamiliar surroundings. It doesn't take much to tip the scale.

As the Alzheimer's progresses, traveling—and even extended outings—may create more stress than enjoyment for both of you. Unfortunately, travelling together will one day become a pleasure of the past. Investing your time and energy into planning and getting through the trip makes little sense if it only results in confusion and conflict.

On one occasion, Marshall and I had a layover in the Denver airport. When he said he had to use the rest room, I stood outside while he went in. As the minutes passed, I became increasingly alarmed that he had not come out. I explained the situation to a gentleman entering the rest room who kindly complied with my request to check on Marshall. He wasn't in there. That's when I realized he had walked out through a second exit.

I tried his cell phone, but he did not answer. I looked up and down the airport concourse but could not find him. After about fifteen minutes of heart-pounding panic I spied him strolling down from the opposite end of the terminal toward me.

I ran down to him dragging all our carry-on baggage and asked where he had been. "Nowhere," he said, and asked with irritation, "Where were you?" I tried to tell him that I was worried about him, that I didn't know where he'd been. But things got very twisted. He yelled at me for wandering away and causing a scene.

Our argument was brought to a halt when an announcement signaled that our flight was boarding. Marshall at first resisted getting on the plane, and, once on, argued about his seat. He wanted to sit toward the front of the plane and wouldn't move down the aisle. I grew increasingly more anxious. I begged him to move along and sit down in our assigned seats. Airlines don't tolerate disruptions, and I was afraid Marshall's behavior would get us thrown off the plane.

Little I said could convince Marshall to comply and shake off his ornery mood—until I remembered I had a chocolate bar in my bag. I told him if he took his assigned seat, he could have it.

And that was it. He went to his seat, sat down, and never said another word about it. He was too busy enjoying his candy.

No matter how much thought we have put into carefully planning an outing or vacation, we have to be ready for a sudden change of plans, perhaps to cancel them all together, or at least to brace ourselves for some rough patches along the way. Keeping this in mind from the start will help us manage the disappointment we might feel if we cannot carry out our original plan. If things repeatedly fizzle after several attempted getaways, it is time to recognize these trips are no longer doable.

✔ WHAT WE CAN DO...

- Make a check list and be sure to carry medications, important documents, a change of clothes, and snacks

when traveling.
- Place contact information in your spouse's pockets, handbag, or wallet.
- Alert TSA agents, flight attendants, and the hotel desk clerks of your spouse's condition.

Our Marital Identity

As married people, we have two identities. We are known individually and as a couple. Part of our attraction to someone is based on this image of how we appear to others, our image as a couple. We are often defined by what we do together, who we help or work with, and how we stand out among our friends and neighbors.

I enjoyed Marshall and I enjoyed our marital identity. We were magical together. We were perceived by everyone we knew as a happy, friendly, and welcoming couple. Our home was open to friends and family at all times and we greeted neighbors on the street with sincerity and kindness.

As Marshall's illness wrought changes in him, our identity as a couple changed. People began to grow cautious in approaching us. We were less able to socialize with our friends. Marshall's larger-than-life personality gradually slipped away. He became anxious and timid. I grew stressed, exhausted, and depressed. And I virtually vanished from several groups I'd previously been active in. I couldn't leave Marshall home alone, and if I brought him with me to some activity, my engagement with the group had to be minimal.

We changed. We are not the couple we once were. Alzheimer's beat us up and wore us down. But we're still here in this Alzheimer's relationship.

I've always been protective of the dignity Marshall is entitled to. He is not just my husband, but a man of great accomplishment. He ran businesses and entertained audiences across the country. I never want him to feel less than the incredible, dynamic man that he is.

He continues to be recognized in public, so I always strive to protect his image as a beloved character. He loved his fans and they loved him right back. There is a charisma about him that continues today. I don't want anything to interfere with that legacy, which he spent his life building.

Until recently, many outsiders had difficulty recognizing Marshall's disability. And it is ironic how close some of these people are to him. From my perspective, Marshall's problems were obvious. But few besides our doctors noticed his decline. Marshall looked outwardly strong and healthy. He is still polite and friendly, and he knows how to shift attention away from his inability to follow a conversation or remember his connection to the people he sees. After all, he is a life-long master of misdirection.

This ability prevents outsiders from understanding how little he remembers of the past or how poorly he comprehends what is said to him now. The risk is that an ill-spoken response from him can come across as rude. The Alzheimer's can make him uncensored, paranoid, and delusional. He can appear uninterested and make thoughtless comments. His hearing is poor, so he can be very loud in declaring his opinions. He doesn't hesitate to announce, "That lady looks fat in that dress."

Such behavior puts me in an awkward position. Outsiders may think I am overbearing in my protection of him. They are unaware of how much Marshall truly needs. I order his food. I speak for him in public. When we still traveled, I guided him through airports and hotels. From the looks of strangers, I know some think it odd for me to be telling this senior gentleman to perform the simplest of actions. On one occasion, a young receptionist in a doctor's office ordered me to stop answering her questions for Marshall and take a seat, which I did. A few minutes later she came over to me and asked if I'd answer her questions. She never apologized for her rudeness, but she very quickly realized Marshall could not do what she asked of him.

✔ WHAT WE CAN DO...

- Concentrate on your needs and your spouse's needs, not on what other people think.
- Know that you are not responsible for your spouse's behavior.
- Remember that your spouse is not really responsible for their actions.

The Big Events

Ironically, close friends and family may not view us with any more compassion or understanding than strangers. The joys of family and friendships are usually celebrated by marking momentous events together. Weddings, landmark birthdays, graduations, personal achievements, and holidays are toasted together by a whole family joined in celebration. They are events we eagerly look forward to, but our spouses with Alzheimer's may find them overwhelming. Even if our spouses says they want to go, anxiety can mount for them in the days leading up to the event. Once there, their energy is quickly drained.

Even close relations cannot understand how much they are asking when they invite Alzheimer's sufferers to their celebration. It's important to them that our loved one is there, but if he or she is in mid-to-late stages of Alzheimer's, all the people and activity at the event will be too much. There is so much to absorb, and those with Alzheimer's are working with too little cognitive ability to process it all. Recovery from such an event will take several days—even though they have no memory of it.

If the event is close by, a preferred alternative to attending the entire celebration is to make a brief appearance. Travel time must be included when considering how much is too much. Limit outings to no more than two or three hours, including travel time, for best results. If the party is too far away to fit that window, it is better to send your regrets.

The best option for Alzheimer's patients is for the person celebrating to come to them for a short visit prior to the event. Commemorative photos can still be taken, and they can have our spouse all to themselves, undistracted and comfortable in a familiar setting. It may be a great disappointment to the extended family that we cannot attend the celebration, but it is better to celebrate in a way that considers our loved one's best interests.

✔ WHAT WE CAN DO...

- Do what is best for you and your spouse even if outsiders don't understand.
- Offer alternative opportunities for family to celebrate with your spouse.
- Try not to let the anger and disappointment of others hurt you.

Tipping the Scale of Responsibility

Marriage is a partnership, a shared relationship. We give and we take. We compromise, committed as we both should be to working together for our mutual good.

Both spouses are expected to care for themselves *and* care for their partner. The necessary level of compromise on each partner's part will vary throughout our lives. In the typical marriage, and in our own expectations, the balance may lean more heavily in one direction at times. Illness, unemployment, financial difficulties, career conflicts...many life events can shift the burden of less-than-willing compliance temporarily. But most often, the period of imbalance is limited.

We know better than to expect to be met halfway on every issue for our entire marriage. We don't even mind giving 100% on some occasions, because our partner is giving back in other areas to such a great degree. It's when one partner regularly fails to pull their share of the load that trouble starts. Such disparity is one of the most common causes of arguments in a marriage. We reasonably expect to work as a team, with each party carrying half of the load, and harbor resentments when we find ourselves bearing an unfair share.

Here is another area where Alzheimer's rocks the boat. The healthy spouse must assume 100% of the responsibility for everything. The house, car, family obligations, finances, investments, legal affairs, and health care for both of us is totally in our hands.

Our spouses are often unable to help with even the most minor chore. Taking out the trash requires them to remember what day to take it out, how to take it out, and where to put it. Mowing the lawn or cooking a pot of soup includes a bewildering series of steps to follow and potentially dangerous tools or utensils.

We sometimes do entrust our spouses with a project to keep them occupied or to make them feel productive. The tools they use must be safe and our close supervision is likely to be needed. And after spending the extra time to help them through the task, we're likely to have to redo it later anyway.

As partners, we used to share the household chores. But now our spouses can't clean a bathroom. They used to manage the bills, but no longer can write a check or balance a checkbook. Evenings consisted of long discussions about the day's events, the nightly news, our career, events in the lives of our friends, but now our spouses have no idea what we are talking about. Not only have we lost those to whom we turned for help in making our own most critical life decisions, we have lost loved ones who previously made many of those decisions by themselves.

And the greater the marital assets, the greater the weight of responsibility now on our shoulders. The big house, properties and other investments, business ventures, children, and grandchildren all need attention. The more we built and acquired together the more we now must take care of completely on our own.

The strength of a rope lies in the intertwining of multiple weaker fibers. It's the same way in marriage. We are at our best when we are bound together in strength. Our ability to help each other begins with our own confidence, talents, and strength, but it is the intertwining of two souls that keeps our marriage strong, that carries us through life's inevitable difficulties.

Alzheimer's forces us to carry our own weight, alone, and to carry our spouse as well. We are but a single, sometimes frizzled, strand. But the strength we find within needs to sustain us both.

In earlier days, Marshall told me that my perseverance and independence were characteristics he admired in me. I was an entity unto myself, with personal interests, talents, goals, and tremendous faith. He knew he never needed to dote on me or worry about me when his fans surrounded him. I could stand on my own two feet with the best of them.

I'm so grateful for that inner strength, the strength that now holds us both up. Still, I wish it didn't have to be this way. Being that single strand in a long, tight rope, bearing a heavy load, is exhausting.

✔ WHAT WE CAN DO...

- Keep projects small. Clean out one drawer, one shelf, one area of the refrigerator.
- If affordable, hire service providers to help with household chores and upkeep our spouse can no longer help with.
- Inquire with church ministries and community organizations about free services and volunteers to help around the house.

Cleaning Up Their Messes

If any of us were to die today, what messes would we leave for our loved ones to clean up? Are our financial and legal affairs in order? What condition are our personal items in? Do we have collections that need to be sold or passed on? Does our family know our wishes on our health, dying, and death?

Most of us have loose ends all over the place. But we have no intention of dying today, so what's the hurry, right? These aren't things that need our immediate attention We're too busy to worry about the distant future.

Here again, Alzheimer's interferes in our marriage and the ability for each partner to address his or her own problems. As I've said earlier, one of the most confounding issues with Alzheimer's sufferers is their inability to recognize their own cognitive decline. Most don't see anything wrong with their sense of reason or decision-making abilities. They don't believe there is any compelling reason to address their affairs. Even if they understand their disease on some level, they're not likely to recognize the urgency of the need to put things in order.

The inevitable consequence is that everything is left for the healthy spouse to handle. And it isn't easy to manage another person's affairs when they are aware we are taking control. Our spouses are adults. They had careers and ran businesses and homes. They may feel we are interfering in their personal affairs and become justifiably angry. They continue to think they are fully capable, and they were already paranoid before we started fiddling with their stuff. Our meddling won't be taken well.

Like so much else about Alzheimer's, we don't want to be in this position of making decisions for them any more than they want us to be doing it. We certainly don't want to use our precious, limited time to clean up the clutter of a lifetime. But some things need to be dealt with now.

This often requires that we act behind our spouses' back, which isn't easy when we are caring for them around the clock. A good marriage is founded on trust. Taking necessary actions we never took without them before can make us feel that we are deceiving them.

If our spouses were working when they began to show symptoms, coworkers and employers may have been the first to notice. Our spouses' personality may have changed from easygoing to quite anxious, agitated, and paranoid, resulting in disagreements with their employer and coworkers, lost business, or other work-related failures. We may need to contact these people to clear up loose ends and rebuild our spouses' hard-earned reputation. .

Neighbors or friends may have been offended by some inappropriate or aggressive behavior. Alzheimer's can make our spouses irritable and uncensored. We may feel the need to make amends for their rude remarks. We don't want the people around us to be hurt. Nor do we want our spouse's good name to be tainted by what they no longer can control.

Unresolved legal issues will have to be attended to. Our own legal affairs are stressful enough, but now we must clear up theirs as well. It is critical that we hold an *enduring* power of attorney (one that continues after their loss of mental capacity). While such instruments are automatically enduring in some states, that is not the case everywhere. Check your own state's policy.

Most of us have accumulated more personal items around our homes and piled in the garage than we will ever use, and now we must care for our spouses' treasures as well as our own. This is one of the most difficult areas to handle because it is obvious when we clean, repair, rearrange, or eliminate items that surround our spouse. So much must be done that we cannot do when our spouse is around. They already feel like everyone is against them. Moving their belongings only agitates them further.

And yet, we are always with them. We have so few moments alone that finding the time to care for our spouse's personal property is nearly impossible.

And there seems to be a never-ending array of medical decisions. Even if we previously had prudent discussions with our spouses about health care, death, and dying, we must now make all the official decisions for them. Would our spouses want to be taking this or that medication? Would they really want a recommended procedure or surgery? How did they feel about medical intervention and death? How did they want their final remains to be handled?

The distribution of their property is another burden that weighs heavily on us. Determining how to distribute personal mementos can be stressful if our spouses have failed to indicate their wishes prior to their illness. Selling off some family treasures may even be necessary to help pay for their care.

We live in a world of countless choices. And now it is up to us to make every single one of them for both our spouse and ourselves. The number of decisions to be made can be among the most tiring and stressful burdens we bear.

✔ WHAT WE CAN DO...

- Make the best decision you can and move on without fussing over whether it was right.
- Take on one issue at a time without worrying about getting everything done immediately.
- Put your own affairs in order.

For Richer or for Poorer

When two people join together in marriage, they commonly join finances. Some couples share equally in bringing in the income as well as caring for the home. Often one spouse is responsible for bringing in the majority of income, perhaps with a job that requires long work hours, while the other cares for the family and home. We're a team working together in a way that works best for the whole.

And, here again is an area we find Alzheimer's disrupting the cooperation of two people in a marriage. Your spouse soon will come to a point when he or she is unable to work and yet is unable to stay home alone while we work. Either you will pay a caregiver to stay home with your spouse while you work, which may not be affordable, or you will stay home with your spouse to care for him or her full-time. The financial burden is staggering either way.

Should we remain home, we not only lose our income but our own future security in pension and social security benefits. This inability to generate income can continue for a decade, sometimes two, indefinitely removing us from the workforce, or at the very least, leaving us at a significant career disadvantage.

Women are the most challenged in this scenario. We are the majority of caregivers, caring for children, parents, and spouses without income a good part of our lives. We often earn less than men, so when women are able to work outside the home, it takes more hours of work to earn the same amount as men. And because of this disparity of wages, we also are paying less into our retirement plan. We end up with a lot less to live on, and for a longer period of time, as women tend to live longer.

Alzheimer's disease is the most expensive disease in the nation. The cost for dementia care in the United States for 2019 is estimated to be $290 billion, a number that could rise as high as 1.1 trillion by 2050. No matter how we care for our spouse with Alzheimer's—whether we care for our spouse ourselves, hire caregivers in our home, or place our spouse into a memory care community—it will cost us dearly.

The cost of a private caregiver for in-home care in the Chicago area where Marshall and I live runs up to $30 an hour at the time of this writing. Costs vary greatly by state, but this is one expense you don't want to skimp on. We need a compassionate caregiver trained to keep our spouses safe as well as to tend to their physical needs. It is critical that caregivers be familiar with dementia care, not just elder care.

Memory care home expenses also vary significantly. Assisted-living facilities that offer memory care averaged $4,400 per month nationally in 2018. However, this fee varies greatly in different areas, and a $5,000 to $11,000 monthly charge is currently more likely in many urban locations.

This is where the foresight in buying long-term care insurance and saving and investing wisely in earlier days pays off. Most long-term care premiums are rapidly increasing, and the policies have per-diem limits, qualify types of coverage, and are limited to a certain length of time. And, be aware that personal savings will also be depleted by expenses not covered under any policy.

Frankly discussing the expense of caring for each other while we are both in good health may seem cold, but it is something that should not be avoided.

✔ WHAT WE CAN DO...

- Speak with a financial advisor as soon as possible.
- Have bills paid automatically to avoid late payments or unpaid bills that may affect your credit.
- Continue saving for your own future as much as possible.

The Legalities

One of the best investments we can make is to hire a good lawyer to execute documents regarding our health and property. An attorney that specializes in elder law can be invaluable in securing our interests over the years ahead.

The earlier we put these documents in place the better. Then we only need to review them periodically for updates. If we don't already have the critical documents at the time of a diagnoses of dementia, it may still be possible to create them. A person with Alzheimer's can execute or update legal documents if the attorney judges them capable of understanding what is involved and making rational decisions.

But time is of the essence in getting these documents completed. We may feel we are strong, healthy, and invincible right now, when the reality is that we can be victims of an accident or disease at any minute. And an illness such as Alzheimer's prevents us from realizing our disability. The moment symptoms begin to surface, recognition of the urgency to act is diminished.

Fortunately, Marshall maintained a relationship with attorneys long before I came into the picture. He regularly made changes and updates to critical documents. I am very grateful to him for keeping on top these documents, because updating them is just as important as initiating them.

Marshall had given me his power of attorney for both medical and property issues before his condition was diagnosed. These documents enabled me to pay his bills, make decisions about his medical care, and access information necessary to care for him. Had he not done so, I may have had to spend a considerable amount of time and incurred serious expense in taking steps necessary to gain control of his affairs.

Marshall's foresight in executing his documents prompted me to get my own affairs in order years ago and to periodically review them. I looked at my documents five years after Marshall was diagnosed with Alzheimer's symptoms and realized that Marshall still held my power of attorney! He was already far beyond the point of being capable of acting on his own behalf, much less mine. I moved quickly to update my designated power of attorney, and now review all my legal documents yearly.

These important documents stipulate who we trust to oversee our health and property in the event we are unable to act on our own behalf. Without proper authorization we cannot make the simplest decisions for our spouse: changing or canceling their cell phone plan, collecting medical records, filing taxes, moving funds, even changing an address on a bank account. Some institutions, such as investment companies and the Social Security Administration, may require their own form of a power of attorney to be completed. But having a notarized power of attorney in hand is the critical first step in getting the others expedited.

The main documents to consider differ slightly state to state, but typically include:

- **Advance Directive for Health Care**—This is a type of power of attorney that names a spouse, domestic partner, close friend, or relative to make medical decisions regarding doctors, health care providers, medical treatments, care facilities, and end of life decisions on our behalf in the event we are incapable of making our own decisions.

- **Advance Directive for Property**—This is a second type of power of attorney that names a spouse, domestic partner, close friend, or relative to make decisions on our behalf regarding our wealth and material goods in the event we are incapable of making our own decision.

- **Living Will**—A Living Will is a type of advance directive that expresses how we wish to be treated in medical situations. This includes a decision about whether we want to receive life support.

- **Standard Will**—This document tells our executor how we wish our property to be distributed after death.

- **Living Trust**—A Living Trust, available in some states, stipulates how our assets will be distributed after death in a way that may avoid probate and offer tax advantages.

Once we do have these documents in place, we should review them yearly or any time our health or financial situations change.

✔ WHAT WE CAN DO...

- Seek out experienced and well-recommended legal and financial advisers.
- If our spouse is capable, have them see an attorney to document their wishes regarding both healthcare and property.
- Ensure that your spouse updates their documents when necessary for as long as they are able.

Be Brave

The constant stream of decisions confronting us requires that we be strong, even courageous. However disheartening they might be, most decisions don't need a lot of thought. But there are so many to make, and so many have serious consequences for our spouse's care, our marriage, our home, and our selves.

How can we encourage our spouses to eat breakfast? Can we afford a new dishwasher? Do we need to prevent our spouses from driving? Should we get a second medical opinion? Is extensive cognitive testing worth the stress it will put our spouses through? Can we entrust their care to strangers?

The good news is that the many decisions, and the work necessary to see those decisions to fruition, do not need to fall on us alone. In fact, we should not let them. The key is finding all manner of service providers in whom we can place our trust with confidence: physicians, attorneys, accountants, housekeepers, painters, plumbers, lawn services....

Public service institutions in our city, county, and faith community may offer assistance. We also can solicit capable friends and family members, especially ones who understand that the end decisions must be ours. Close relatives often feel that their advice should be followed exactly. We can usually expect to encounter a few unsolicited advisors who freely offer suggestions that we know will not help.

Only we know the whole story—what taking a particular course of action may mean to our spouse, and to us. We and our spouse alone share this bond, this Alzheimer's marriage, our long, storied, intimate, once happy, now challenging years together. Only we know what was said and agreed upon between us and even things left unsaid but expected.

Regardless of any advisor's superior expertise, we have the responsibility to make the final decision. We have an obligation to ourselves and our spouse to do our homework, use our head and our heart, but in the end to trust our gut and summon the courage to make the decision. And then don't look back. In hindsight (and in second guessing, I'm afraid) it is so easy to find clarity, a luxury we don't enjoy in the present moment. With all we have on our plates, we can barely see what's in front of us today, much less where it is going to take us tomorrow. We can only make the best decision we can and accept in our hearts the certain knowledge that we have done our best.

✔ WHAT WE CAN DO...

- Consult with a trusted close friend or family member.
- Rely on what is in your own heart and mind to make decisions.
- Remember that outsiders, however well intended, have no rights to make final decisions for you.

Love and Honor All the Days of My Life

Marshall and I complemented each other. He coaxed me out my shell and into a more public life, and I brought him a home, dinner on the table, family time, and quiet evenings. For many years we traveled extensively and enjoyed the company of friends. We worked side-by-side from home offices and on magic shows. Neither of us cared to waste time on petty arguments. We shared a peaceful, gentle, and happy relationship.

In many ways, I believe that our early years together helped to prepare us for what was to come. Before we were married, Marshall ate nearly all of his meals in restaurants. He was out every night, visiting friends, working shows, and attending performances. After we married, he discovered the comforts of home. He frequently thanked me for the home-cooked meals he came to enjoy. We watched movies and television together in the evenings in what became a sanctuary for both of us. We shared the joys and comforts of a beautiful home with friends and family regularly.

By the time he could no longer work, he was accustomed to spending his days with me. He didn't mind that I drove when he could not. He trusted me and my decisions.

I also changed because of him. Marshall was an avid traveler and taught me how to maneuver through airports and hotels. His back seat driving annoyed me, but I must admit he helped make me a better driver. Household finances and maintenance of the home were my responsibilities from the beginning. If I told him I wanted to make some change, he encouraged me to go for it. He made me feel strong and independent. By the time Marshall developed Alzheimer's, I was already comfortable running the home, acting as our driver, assisting him with magic shows, and planning our travel. These were things I'd always done.

And we were content being together all the time. At the beginning of our marriage, Marshall asked me to quit my job in advertising, which I did. His work schedule as a consultant was flexible, and he was anxious that we enjoy together the freedom to attend magic conventions, travel, and meet with his many out-of-town friends.

The timing to step out of the workforce and venture away from home wasn't the best for me. I had three young teenagers to watch out for and was building a writing career. My mother was diagnosed with cancer the year after our wedding and I needed and wanted to assist with her care and my father's adjustment to their changing situation.

My mother only lived three years after her diagnosis, and then my father developed cancer. I cared for him as much as I could until he passed away three years after my mother. Within six years, both of my parents were gone at the relatively young ages of 70 and 74.

Combining my family obligations with all the travel Marshall wanted to do required considerable juggling. But I don't regret a moment of that busy time. Marshall began showing symptoms of Alzheimer's only two years after my father passed away. Had I waited until my parents were gone and the kids were grown, I'd have experienced significantly less time alone with Marshall. We continued to travel and do shows for several years after he was diagnosed, but doing so began to require such extensive planning and maneuvering that it became more stressful than enjoyable for me. Still, I remain grateful to this day for the opportunities we had to be together.

✔ WHAT WE CAN DO...

- Think back on the ways your life prepared you for this journey.
- Recognize the inner strength that you developed before Alzheimer's became a part of your life.
- Do your best to enjoy all aspects of your life.

Slipping Away

From the beginning of our marriage, Marshall liked to sleep. He rose late in the morning, napped in the afternoon, and fell asleep in his chair by early evening. Over the years the ratio of awake time to sleep time continued to shift toward the sleep side. I attributed his need for rest to aging, but Alzheimer's may already have been wearing him down. The disease was likely attacking brain cells long before our wedding day, possibly for as long as a decade.

As Alzheimer's disease progresses, our loved ones consume energy just trying to process simple daily activities and whatever is happening around them. They have less and less brain power to work with. Pausing throughout the day for a short respite increasingly becomes more of a necessity. Our spouses need to stop and recharge often.

Their moments of withdrawal forewarn us of what is to come. First, it's later risings, frequent naps, and early bedtimes. Parties progressively end earlier. Vacations become shorter.

And then the emotional detachment starts. Maybe they grow irritable. Our special moments are intermixed with strange reactions and hurtful comments. Our spouses becomes less sensitive to us and our needs. They begin withdrawing from our friends and extended family, and finally us.

Gradually, they retreat into a silent world wholly within. Other people fade from their mind. One by one, we are forgotten. Knowing it isn't their fault makes it no less painful. We long for the spouse we married and the deep love we shared.

Marshall never formally asked me to marry him. I felt cheated of that singular moment of proposal for decades. He told me on our first date that we should marry and asked often if I wanted to be with him. But he never spoke the words I wanted so much to hear, "Mary, will you marry me?"

In all honesty, he may not have been able to get down on one knee comfortably: he was sixty when we decided to get married. Nor would he have. Marshall had never been the romantic type. It just wasn't in him to plan an elaborate and memorable proposal.

What is so ironic about that lack of formal proposal now is that nearly every day through the years that Marshall has had Alzheimer's disease, he's asked me to marry him. He forgets that we are married and has often been delighted to learn that we are.

It's too late for any attempt by Marshall to get down on one knee. Alzheimer's has robbed him of physical abilities as well as mental ones. In any event, I treasure every "I love you" and every proposal he offers me now as I realize these too will fade.

Caregivers and Alzheimer's medical providers often predicted that Marshall would always maintain that emotional connection. Long after he had forgotten who I was, he'd feel safe with me. He'd always welcome my close presence.

I'm not so sure about their promise any longer. Although I often find Marshall to be content, the days when I cannot connect with him on any level are growing. Some days he is totally lost to me.

✔ WHAT WE CAN DO...

- We need to rest when our spouse rests. The tasks of the day can wait and we will feel better.
- Savor the moments our spouse does connect with us.
- Acknowledge the sorrow when our spouse does not recognize us. It is a loss better mourned than denied.

Close but Not Intimate

By mid-to-late Alzheimer's, we must manage most of our spouses' daily needs—bathing, dressing, and feeding them. Most likely, though, sexual intimacy is part of our past. Our roles have changed, and naturally so have our feelings. We are a caregiver and they are the care receiver.

Yes, we are spouses. We're still married. But we aren't partners. We don't share decisions and responsibilities. Because of this, it isn't unusual for our feelings to change. The caregiving role has altered our passions. Alzheimer's changed us both, and therefore, our relationship.

Alzheimer's sufferers' sexual drive and physical ability to perform can be adversely affected by the disease and any number of medications they may be taking. Failed attempts at sexual intimacy can frustrate both spouses.

And if one spouse does not recognize the other as such, either or both may even believe intimacy is inappropriate. Advances may frighten them. It's not uncommon for a wife of many decades to object to her husband seeing her undressed or to sleeping in her bed. She may not remember that they are married, and often doesn't remember her husband at all.

Other couples continue to sleep in the same bed and cuddle. For them, the physical contact is comforting. And in a world where our spouse can be frightened in their own home, they may feel safer close to us at night. Still, sexual advances may not be of interest to either party.

There are no rules in the Alzheimer's marriage. How physically close we get is a personal choice. Whatever is most comfortable for both spouses is best for the couple.

As with all areas of our marriage, things change as our spouses progress through the later stages of Alzheimer's. What works today may not work tomorrow. Some loved ones may remain affectionate for some time, while others progressively become less so. Our Alzheimer's spouses' behavior can change, often within a few hours, and so will their preferences regarding intimacy. There isn't any perfect way to predict how any of this will go.

Since he first began to experience symptoms of Alzheimer's, Marshall has acquired the habit of holding my hand, not something we did previously. He was always in a hurry, and I didn't move along fast enough for him. He wanted me close but not physically touching in public.

Currently, he doesn't care who hears his affectionate words to me or sees his desire to be physically close. Partly because of his diminished ability to hear, he shouts how he loves me and that I'm the love of his life.

Although Alzheimer's has long ago destroyed the traditional intimacy we once shared, we enjoy a new type of closeness that feels appropriate at this point in our lives. We treasure hugs and hand-holding. My heart still flutters when I'm in his arms. Together, we are at peace.

Finding our new normal under difficult situations is what makes us unique as a couple. We may no longer enjoy the passionate love of newlyweds, but our relationship can be beautiful and tender in its own way.

✔ WHAT WE CAN DO...

- Enjoy the new intimacy of holding hands and snuggling on the couch.
- Sleep in another room if your spouse is uncomfortable with you in their bed.
- Remember that it is Alzheimer's that has interfered with your sex life, not your spouse.

When We're Physically Separated

For many reasons, in any marriage, we can find ourselves separated from our partner. Work, mental and physical illnesses, military service, imprisonment, and marital differences can force us apart. Every scenario brings with it its own trials. Such separations put grave stress on the relationship and each party individually. In our loved one's absence, we face loneliness, resentment, longing, and depression.

Alzheimer's is one cause of physical separation. The healthy spouse may no longer be able to provide the care their loved one needs. Or the home may no longer be safe for our spouse. The best option at this time is for our spouse to move to a memory care community.

Early in Marshall's disease I was often asked what my plans were. Would I move him to a home for Alzheimer's, and if so when? My response was that I hoped not. I prayed that I could keep him in our home until the very end.

For many years I believed I could achieve that goal. As stressful as it was, I wanted my husband to stay home with me. I thought that he would be devastated by moving to a strange new home, living among strangers.

Unfortunately, we reached a point where keeping Marshall at home was no longer safe or healthy for either one of us. After caring for him myself for ten years, I admitted that I could no longer care for him alone. Marshall was wandering out the door and falling down stairs. He became agitated with workers around the house. It was difficult to keep dangerous items out of his hands. He experienced episodes of unwarranted aggression and rage.

I was rapidly losing weight and developing multiple illnesses. The 24/7 caregiving responsibilities wore me out. Endless days and nights of vigilance and the tremendous responsibility of caring for an adult man who was no longer able to care for himself were breaking me. Yet I resisted moving him for far too long.

Our family physician had encouraged me to place Marshall in a memory care community for at least three years before I finally agreed. As the doctor said, Marshall needed a team of people working around the clock to assist him, and while I would continue to care for him it would be as a part of that team. While relinquishing much of my responsibilities to a qualified staff, I could oversee his care without doing the constant hands-on work, return to my role as wife, regain my own sanity and physical health, with the hope of spending our time together enjoying each other's presence.

But the relief of the 24/7 care did not come without a price—and not just the monetary one. We suddenly went from being together every minute of every day to having daily visits. The transition for Marshall was difficult, but he adapted to the change more quickly than I did. He continued to ask for me and was happy when we were together, but he also became quickly acclimated to his new community.

I, on the other hand, went into deep depression. This was a change I had fought off for years. I felt defeated. I was lonesome for my husband. My sense of purpose took a downward spiral.

Marshall had been my daily obsession. Everything I did all day long, all night long, was for him, and now he was in more capable hands, and he easily accepted what I feared he would reject. I felt I had been replaced.

Marshall and I continue to long for the way things were before Alzheimer's insinuated itself into our marriage. We miss sharing our entire days and evenings. Perhaps, though, the greatest loss for both of us occurs with nightfall. Those leisure evenings watching television together and snuggling at bedtime are so sorely missed.

✔ WHAT WE CAN DO...

- Consider moving your spouse to assisted living for memory care before the home environment becomes unsafe.
- After a move to assisted living, enjoy your reprised role as spouse and comforter rather than full-time caregiver.
- Remember that nothing can replace your spousal love.

Faithful Unto You

Marriage hangs, above all else, on our agreement to be true to one another. We made a covenant, an agreement to be faithful. Even showing affection for another person can be damaging to a marriage. Our intimate affections should exclusively be for our spouse.

Here again, Alzheimer's messes with everything we believe in. Our spouses' sense of reasoning is diminished, if not completely gone. If they are in a memory-care home or a day-care setting, they may form bonds with new partners. Our spouses don't understand the marriage agreement anymore. They may not even be aware that they are married. And neither will their new friend.

Marshall had a couple of girlfriends in his home. It wasn't unusual for me to find him holding hands with one of them, heads together, even exchanging intimate words. Most often, he would turn away from his friend when I entered and was eager to go off with me. Other times he needed to be pried away.

Encountering Marshall with a girlfriend was awkward for me for several reasons. He was with those women most of the day. They needed companionship and didn't understand normal boundaries. I felt bad about breaking them up. I didn't want to hurt the ladies' feelings. But I do admit that, as much as I understood the situation, it hurt me every time.

In my efforts to ease everyone through the situation, I would happily greet them both and talk with them for a while, then ask Marshall if he'd like to walk with me. When he got up, I would tell his lady friend I would bring him back to her. I would try to offer another friend to sit near her or ask a caregiver to engage her while we were gone.

Our feelings about other potential partners can be tested as well. How do we stay true to our spouse when he or she is unavailable to us on every level for so many years? We need intimacy. We're healthy and longing for passion. Are we unfaithful if we seek comfort in another person? These are deeply personal issues and decisions we alone can make.

- Remember that, although Alzheimer's masks it, the love your spouse had for you, and still has, doesn't end.
- Ask a caregiver to separate your spouse from their friend before your expected arrival.
- Acknowledge your feelings and talk about them with friends or a counselor.

Who Takes Care of Us?

How often are we told by a well-meaning friend to be sure to take care of ourselves? Every time I hear the phrase, it feels like a joke. Few seem to grasp the all-consuming amount of responsibility weighing down on us. Our workload is beyond manageable. Intellectually, we know what they're saying—that we must care for ourselves—is true but figuring out how in the world to do that is challenging. The thought of taking time off is not at all realistic. Alzheimer's does not take a vacation.

But however difficult it seems to be, caring for ourselves truly needs to be among our highest priorities. The best way to justify self-care is to recognize how difficult life would be for our spouse if something happened to us. Caring for ourselves is meeting a responsibility to them, not a selfish gesture. If we grow too run down to keep up the difficult pace, or become ill, or pass away, we can't care for our spouse any longer. Other family members will suffer, as they will need to step in. Neglecting our own well being will leave us of use to no one. I know this to be true from personal experience.

Many years ago, a friend expressed her frustration about reaching her senior years without getting "her day." She supported her children and husband her whole married life, and she always did so with great joy. But she also felt she'd lost the opportunity to express herself along the way. She asked, "Mary, when is it my turn?"

My response was, "When you take it."

Like most people, I'm fabulous at offering excellent advice that I don't follow myself. My health has suffered greatly from the relentless onslaught of sleep deprivation, stress, and heartache over all these years. I didn't call in assistance soon enough, or periodically step away as I now realize I should have. We caregivers are drowning in the turbid ocean of Alzheimer's responsibilities, and I've learned the hard way that the only lifesaver that will come our way is the one we create.

Family caregivers to a loved one with dementia experience higher levels of psychological distress than caregivers of any other illnesses. Such caregivers report a significantly higher number of health problems than non-caregivers. We are at increased risk of depression, anxiety, cardiovascular problems, lower immunity, poor sleep patterns, slower wound healing, diabetes, arthritis, ulcers, and anemia.

Employers are expected to provide full-time employees with breaks through the day, to define specified work hours, and to offer a periodic vacation. Even God took a day's rest. Jesus rested. How can we imagine we don't need rest as well?

My counselor once asked me why I thought Marshall's life was more valuable than my own. I responded that it was because he needed my undivided attention. He couldn't take care of himself. She pointed out that I didn't answer her question.

If I have learned anything from my many conversations with other Alzheimer's spouses, it is that my situation is common. We give 100% of ourselves to our spouses and forget the importance of caring for our own needs. Fear of leaving our spouses in un-qualified hands, the desire to be with them, the belief that we are obligated to attend to their every need ourselves, are all among the reasons we think we cannot step away.

Even after placing a spouse in a memory-care community, our sense of obligation and devotion do not end. We continue to be with our loved one as often as possible. Phone calls from him or her and the staff, particularly at odd hours, alarm us. Authorization of medical treatment and other changes in care remain our responsibility. And we continue to take them to countless appointments, a task that, like everything else we experience with Alzheimer's, becomes progressively more difficult.

✓ WHAT WE CAN DO...

- Take a break and meet with friends once or twice a week.
- If your spouse is still at home, place him or her in respite care for a week or two every six months so you can take a restorative vacation.
- Keep in mind that caring for yourself is caring for your spouse.

Making Healthy Choices

We hear repeatedly of the importance of exercising regularly and maintaining a healthy diet. Finding the time to do either is challenging while we're deep into caregiving, but we—especially—must not forget their importance. We need the nourishment, and the exercise burns off the stress as well as helping to keep us physically fit. A good night's sleep is vital as well, however difficult this may be to accomplish without assistance through the night.

Scheduling time off daily, weekly, and seasonally is essential to our well being. I know from my own mistakes how damaging it is to not step away for a day, an hour, a moment of self-care. Periodic breaks throughout the day might include a cup of tea or coffee, listening to relaxing music, playing a musical instrument, praying, getting lost in a good book or movie, or taking a walk for fresh air and sunshine. Even a well-timed fifteen-minute break can be rejuvenating.

Opportunities for respite can be created by eliminating unnecessary housework, gardening, and other projects. Selling, giving away, or discarding household items not really needed will leave you with fewer items to clean and provide more opportunities for small breaks. A smaller home, and perhaps one that includes outside maintenance and lawn care services, will lessen the amount of time you need to spend on chores. Cooking simpler meals will reduce the amount of time you must spend in the kitchen. Whatever you can do to simplify cleaning, maintaining the home, and food preparation will open up your schedule and help prevent a dangerous burnout.

Numerous studies prove the importance of socializing to our mental health. We need to get out and converse with peers. The intellectual stimulation and companionship are necessary and beneficial on many levels. I am not saying that this is easy. Finding opportunities for low-stress social interaction can be a considerable challenge, and the looming specter of an absent spouse can make social situations feel awkward as well.

We spouses find ourselves in a rather unique social position. We don't quite fit any conventional category. We aren't divorced or widowed, something people are accustomed to. We are married but strangely alone. We may find ourselves feeling uncomfortable when out with a group of married people. And our single friends have every right to seek a new romantic connection on a Saturday night. Since we aren't interested in finding one ourselves, being with them while they explore possibilities can make us quite uncomfortable.

For me, it's easier to meet friends for lunch. That time of day itself tends to be more relaxed. If I venture out on the weekends, it's usually with family. That's the time I reserve to catch up with my siblings, children, and grandchildren.

Support groups offer us opportunities to socialize in a unique way—engaging with people who have walked in our shoes. Meeting family caregivers who truly understand what we're going through can be beneficial to us, and hearing about our experience can be beneficial to everyone there. These groups are havens where we can honestly vent our concerns, share our good experiences, and gain tips from other caregivers. We can speak openly without fear of judgment. Consulting with counselors or clergy is a good option if we wish to express ourselves more privately.

In addition, when we move a spouse to a memory care facility, we meet others who share our situation. Although no two stories are the same, the havoc Alzheimer's wreaks in our marriages is similar. We share that common intruder. Other spouses can give us guidance and support in a way no one else can. Few outsiders fathom our pain.

If our spouse lives in a memory-care community, the caregivers there can provide us with support and guidance as well. They not only understand and care for our spouse, their knowledge, expertise, and sense of caring are also available to us. These are people we can talk to openly about the down-and-dirty realities of Alzheimer's. Little we can tell them, or our spouse can do, will surprise these compassionate, dedicated, and hardworking people.

✔ WHAT WE CAN DO...

1. Take brief breaks throughout the day, every day.

2. Meet with a friend at least once a week.

3. Never minimize the importance of caring for yourself.

What Others Can Do for Us

Alzheimer's is too monstrous an opponent for anyone to face alone. We're drowning in responsibility and have to ask for help if we are to survive it. So many of us do not. Thirty percent of caregivers die before the spouse they are caring for. Calling on family or friends to contribute to our loved one's care, inquiring if volunteers are available at our church or in our community, or hiring a caregiver to regularly relieve us is essential for not just our own well being but ultimately for that of our spouse. It is important for us to delegate as much as possible. Doing so will avoid depleting our energy. If we are lucky enough to have people who are ready and willing to pitch in, we should take advantage of it.

Keeping a "Yes, You Can Help!" list handy will keep tasks that can be delegated to volunteers and close family members at your fingertips. When someone offers casually, "Let me know if I can do anything," whip out the list and let them choose something they'd like to do.

If a neighbor is running to the store and asks if they can pick anything up for us, we can quickly check the list and tell them what we need. If one of our children, other family members, or close friends visit, we can ask them to bring a healthy, home-cooked meal, mow the lawn, fix a leaky faucet, or stay with our loved one for an hour or two so we can get a haircut. In the best scenario, they will offer to take these tasks on permanently, and we can scratch the item from our list.

At the end of the day, what we need most may be something as simple as a friend's compassion, friendship, and a nonjudgmental ear. Remind friends that we love to spend time with them. We appreciate them not giving up on our friendship, and their patience in accepting the scattered opportunities that arise to see them.

I'm grateful for my many friends who waited for me while I was sunken in the depths of Alzheimer's care with Marshall. Now that he has an entire team of caregivers, I can once again find time for important friendships. The first year or so that Marshall was in the memory care community, he often said he was concerned for me because all I did was work and see him. He reminded me that he was surrounded by new friends, enjoying a range of activities throughout the day. He encouraged me to get out and see my friends too. Even in his diminished capacity, he showed more insight about my well-being than I possessed myself.

✔ WHAT WE CAN DO...

1. Don't be afraid to speak up for what you need.

2. Ask family members to take over responsibility for a particular task.

3. Make a practice of getting out on your own once or twice a week.

Where Does It Leave Us?

Happiness is a choice, in many ways. There's beauty, love, and support around us. We only have to reach out and grasp it. We find ourselves in the midst of what is almost certainly the most trying time of our marriage. When we are exhausted and frustrated, it can be easy to overlook the small joys in our life—the joys both within and beyond our spouse. If we must live with hardship, we should also enjoy these gifts.

My life, no doubt like yours, has been a continuous mix of struggles and blessings. I've had my share of financial hardship, physical illness, chronic pain, loneliness through dark nights, irrational fears, unhelpful personal confrontations... Most often, these difficulties run concurrent with the love, compassion, and support of friends, family, coworkers, and even strangers. To ignore these rich gifts that come our way is a mistake. Why should we dwell in darkness?

Perhaps the most important thing we can do is to get rest. Stop throughout the day, take a nap when our spouse naps if we were up all night, and get to bed at a reasonable hour. The world is a rosier place after a good night's sleep.

And we should never lose sight of the role we are now playing in our marriage. We are living out our vows to the extreme as we care for a loved one who is unable to care for himself or herself. We are giving of ourselves physically, emotionally, and spiritually in the best way we possibly can. We are keeping the most important promise we ever made.

There will come a point, if we outlive our spouse, when the ordeal will be over. There's no telling now just how that will feel. We've been suspended in perpetual loss, spinning each day in a continuous cycle of decline. We're always mourning a part of our spouse, a part of our marriage, that has just been lost. Will the end of such gradual loss serve to make the acceptance of his or her death somehow easier?

Perhaps our loved one's death will bring relief, an end to seeing him or her in such a diminished state, particularly if the last days are difficult. But no doubt, there will be another type of mourning. We will have been so invested in caring for our spouses, often for years or even decades. All the energy we have spent worrying about and caring for them will need to find a new direction. We will have lost one of the most important jobs of our lives.

Until that day, let's vow to enjoy the little things that make our marriage and our life as a whole so wonderful, the special God-given gifts of grace we've received.

And once again, let me remind you that I hold you close in prayer.

✔ WHAT WE CAN DO...

- Don't wait for a better day. Enjoy what you have with your spouse now before it is gone as well.
- Forgive yourself for impatience.
- Don't dwell on past decisions you may now wish you had made differently.
- List your many blessings as a reminder of the positive things in your life.
- Take a moment every day to imagine yourself, as I do, in the embrace of the millions of men and women who share our experience of somehow finding the grace to keep our promise to our spouse.

Acknowledgments

Marriage is difficult under the best of circumstances in our busy, turbulent world. I've been fortunate to witness so many marriages that exemplify the give and take we expect to find in healthy partnerships. Marriages vary as much as the individuals in them, but love and respect are the constants that keep them alive.

In recent years I have also encountered couples, like my husband and me, who struggle under the duress of Alzheimer's disease. Alzheimer's stresses every facet of married life. Couples do the best they can as they continuously adjust their partnerships to the downward spiral of the disease.

I am very grateful to the countless spouses who've shared their stories, their very personal challenges in dealing with Alzheimer's. I thank them for allowing me a peek into these very special relationships.

My team of first reviewers also has my gratitude. Patricia Brewer, Erin Lukasiewicz, and Susan Holstein are dependable readers of all my manuscripts. I'm thankful for this dedicated group who add so much to my work.

I'm also very grateful to Pam Sebern for reading this manuscript as she read *Navigating Alzheimer's,* my earlier book on the subject. Her insight as director of a memory care home was invaluable. I'm blessed to call her friend and mentor.

Editors and publishers Mike Coyne and Greg Pierce are not only experienced editors but good, kind men who are sympathetic to an audience I hold dear to my heart. I'm very thankful for the opportunities and expertise they've provided me.

Most of all, I'm blessed to have an extensive circle of loving, supportive family members and friends. They hold me up every day. This journey would be so much more stressful without them and my unwavering faith in a loving God.

Resources

Administration on Aging

330 Independence Ave, S.W.
Washington, DC 20201
https://acl.gov/

Alzheimer's Association

225 North Michigan Avenue, 17th Floor
Chicago, IL 60601
1-800-272-3900
www.alz.org

Alzheimer's Disease Education and Referral Center (ADEAR)

PO Box 8250
Silver Spring, MD 20907
1-800-438-4380
https://www.nia.nih.gov/health/alzheimers

Consumer Consortium on Assisted Living

www.ccal.org
703-533-8121

Alzheimer's Foundation of America (AFA)

322 8th Avenue, 7th Floor
New York, NY 10001
1-866-AFA-8484 (1-866-232-8484)
www.alzfdn.org

Caregiver Acton Network

1150 Connecticut Ave NW
Suite 501
Washington D.C. 20036
202-454-3970
www.caregiver.action.org

Financial Planning Association (FPA)

Denver, CO; Washington, DC
1-800-322-4237
www.fpanet.org

Medicare

Hotline: 1-800-633-4227
www.medicare.gov

National Adult Day Services Association (NADSA)

1421 E. Broad Street
Suite 425
Fuquay-Varina, NC 27526
877-745-1440
www.nadsa.org

National Association of Area Agencies on Aging (n4a)

1730 Rhode Island Avenue, NW,
Suite 1200
Washington, DC 20036
1-202-872-0888
www.n4a.org

National Association of Professional Geriatric Care Managers (GCM)

3275 West Ina Road
Suite 130
Tucson, AZ 85741
1-520-881-8008
http://www.aginglifecare.org/ALCA/Home

National Eldercare Locator

1-800-677-1116
Eldercare.gov/eldercare.net/public/index.aspx

National Hospice and Palliative Care Organization (NHPCO)

1731 King St
Alexandria, VA 22314
1-703-837-1500
www.nhpco.org

Social Security Administration

1-800-772-1213
www.ssa.gov

Books from In Extenso Press

AFTER THE FEAR COME THE GIFTS: Breast Cancer's Nine Surprising Blessings, by Kay Metres

ALL THINGS TO ALL PEOPLE: A Catholic Church for the Twenty-First Century, by Louis DeThomasis, FSC

THE ALZHEIMER'S SPOUSE: Finding the Grace to Keep the Promise, by Mary K. Doyle

BAPTIZED FOR THIS MOMENT: Rediscovering Grace All Around Us, by Stephen Paul Bouman

CATHOLIC BOY BLUES: A Poet's Journey of Healing, by Norbert Krapf

CATHOLIC WATERSHED: The Chicago Ordination Class of 1969 and How They Helped Change the Church, by Michael P. Cahill

CHRISTIAN CONTEMPLATIVE LIVING: Six Connecting Points, by Thomas M. Santa, CSSR

DEATH IN CHICAGO: WINTER: A Cosmo Grande Murder Mystery, by Dominic J. Grassi

GREAT MEN OF THE BIBLE: A Guide for Guys, by Martin Pable, OFM Cap

THE GROUND OF LOVE AND TRUTH: Reflections on Thomas Merton's Relationship with the Woman Known as "M," by Suzanne Zuercher, OSB

HOPE: One Man's Journey of Discovery from Tormented Child to Social Worker to Spiritual Director, by Marshall Jung

MASTER OF CEREMONIES and **UNDER PAIN OF MORTAL SIN:** Two Bryn Martin Murder Mysteries, by Donald Cozzens

NAVIGATING ALZHEIMER'S: 12 Truths about Caring for Your Loved One, by Mary K. Doyle

PISTACO: A Tale of Love in the Andes, by Lynn F. Monahan

SHRINKING THE MONSTER: Healing the Wounds of Our Abuse, by Norbert Krapf

THE SILENT SCHISM: Healing the Serious Split in the Catholic Church, by Louis DeThomasis, FSC, and Cynthia A. Nienhaus, CSA

THE UNPUBLISHED POET: On Not Giving Up on Your Dream, by Marjorie L. Skelly

WAYWARD TRACKS: Revelations about fatherhood, faith, fighting with your spouse, surviving Girl Scout camp…, by Mark Collins

WE THE (LITTLE) PEOPLE, artwork by ISz

YOUR SECOND TO LAST CHAPTER: Creating a Meaningful Life on Your Own Terms, by Paul Wilkes

AVAILABLE FROM BOOKSELLERS OR 800-397-2282
OR WWW.ACTAPUBLICATIONS .COM